10,000 STEPS
A DAY TO YOUR
OPTIMAL WEIGHT

WALK YOUR WAY TO BETTER HEALTH

10 09 08 07 06   1 2 3 4 5

Library of Congress Cataloging-in-Publication Data

Isaacs, Greg, 1961-
  10,000 steps a day to your optimal weight : walk your way to better health / by Greg Isaacs.
     p. cm.
  ISBN 1-56625-287-3
  1. Fitness walking. 2. Weight loss. 3. Physical fitness. I. Title.
  RA781.65.I83 2006
  613.7'176--dc22
                              2006000397

Cover and Interior Design: Joy Jacob

Volt Press
9255 Sunset Blvd., #711
Los Angeles, CA 90069
www.voltpress.com

CONTENTS

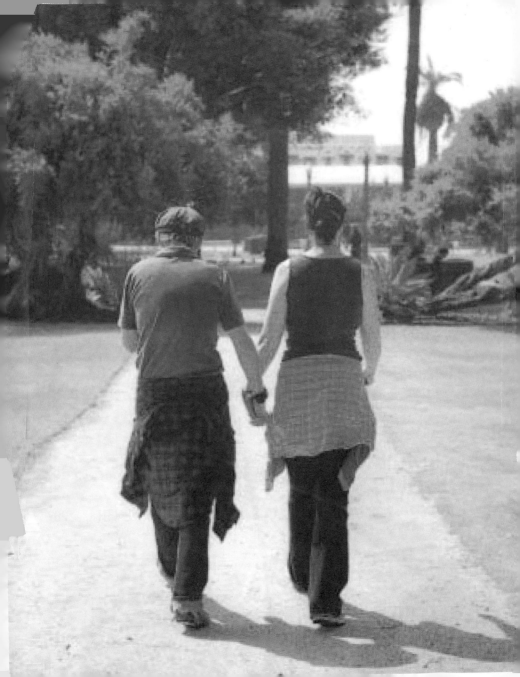

CHAPTER ONE

MAKING THE COMMITMENT

Your First Step to a Trimmer, Healthier You

Congratulations! You've just taken the first and most important step toward ensuring your optimal weight and better health—making the commitment to do something about it. The fact that you're reading this book means you've given serious thought to your physical fitness (and perhaps that of your family and friends too), you've recognized the need and desire to improve your health, and you've decided to take action. Whether your aim is to feel and look better, or to live longer and healthier, or to trim down and tone up, or to replace a high-impact workout with a gentler one, or to mix up your exercise routine by adding an enjoyable new activity you can do virtually any time, anywhere—or all of the above—you've made a wise choice. Because the 10,000-Steps-A-Day Program is based on the most natural, simple, easy, flexible, and effective activity in the world—walking … putting one foot in front of the other, step by step, by 10,000 steps a day.

Right about now, if you're like most people about to try something new, the little naysayer inside is probably peppering you with questions: 10,000 steps? A day? Every day? Right away? Just how far is a walk of 10,000 steps? Do I have to take them all at once? How long will that take? And what do you mean by a "step"? Long step? Short step? Fast step? Slow step? Whoa! Hold on! It's not that complicated. In fact, it's downright simple, as second-nature as … well, walking, which is what the human body is designed for. Plus, this book and the easy-to-use step-counter included with it give you everything you need to count how many steps a day you currently take, just going about your daily life, and how to increase your daily steps gradually and incrementally, based on your fitness level, fitness goals, and lifestyle. It's simply a matter of adding 100 steps here and 1,000 steps there, working toward (or as close as you can and wish to get to) the optimal 10,000 steps a day that, according to the U.S. Surgeon General, the average American needs to maintain weight and improve health. And if you've got the will, the 10,000-Steps-A-Day Program will show you the way—step by step.

What is a step, you ask? A step is simply lifting your leg and placing it down in front of you. It's what you take toward a crying child and toward the people you love when you see them get off an airplane. It's what you take away from a steep ledge or a growling dog. It's what you take when you vacuum the carpet, shop in the mall, and mow the lawn. It's what you take to get from your house to your car and from your car to the grocery store or your workplace. It's also what a golfer takes to line up for a put, a lineman takes

FitnessFACT
It Just Gets Easier

The National Weight Control Registry reports that about 4,500 adults (age 18 and older) who have lost at least 30 pounds and kept it off for at least a year routinely expend about 400 calories a day exercising, with walking being the most frequently used activity. 42% of those participants say that maintaining their weight loss has been less difficult than initially losing it.

when the ball is snapped, and a tennis player takes before swinging the racket. And it's what millions of Americans do for recreation and increasingly for exercise.

Each step is a physical activity requiring the use of multiple muscles working together, and each step consumes energy in the form of calories. Every movement your body makes—from taking a shower to cleaning house to fidgeting—burns calories. In fact, every function your body performs—from digesting to breathing to sleeping—consumes energy. A healthy body requires (and uses) 1 to 1.5 calories per minute just to maintain its "resting" (involuntary) functions, or roughly 10 calories per pound of body weight per day. This basal metabolic rate, or BMR, varies from person to person (and sometimes from day to day), depending on multiple factors, including age, body type, diet, genetics, gender, disease/illness, muscle mass versus fat content, and the body's normal activity level. And active people tend to have higher BMRs than inactive people. But with the 10,000-Steps-A-Day Program, you don't need to worry about your BMR. Just keep in mind that you burn 70-90 calories an hour, or 1680-2160 a day, doing absolutely nothing—and the only way to use up any additional calories is with physical activity.

" If you want to look better [and] feel better, you lower your calorie intake, you lower your fat [and] your carbs, you eat more fruits and vegetables and whole grains, and you exercise—and that's as simple as it can be. "

—Tommy Thomson, U.S. Health and Human Services Secretary

Remember, every movement you make is a physical activity that consumes energy. Even the effortless, mindless act of chewing gum burns 11 calories an hour. A 150-pound person burns about 100 calories walking one mile. A mile is about 2,000 steps. Half a mile, which most people can walk in 10 minutes, is about 1,000 steps. The average American adult takes 900 to 3,000 steps a day going about their normal daily activities; moderately active people take 4,000 to 6,000 steps a day; active people take 10,000-15,000 steps a day. Studies have shown that adding 2,000 steps a day (that's one 20-minute or two 10-minute walks a day) and consuming 100 fewer calories per day (that's a single pat of butter) reduces your risk of heart disease, stroke, diabetes, hypertension, and other chronic diseases; slows down the aging process; improves your mental outlook; and helps you manage your weight and overall health.

Good to Know

In 2001, the U.S. Department of Health and Human Services

published an eye-opening report titled, "The Surgeon General's Call to Action to Prevent and Decrease Overweight and Obesity. This landmark study examined the health risks and costs of the sedentary lifestyles—and resultant weight gains—of an alarming number of Americans. Subsequent government and private studies have revealed that this national health crisis is increasing—but can be corrected by making relatively simple changes to our daily routines.

Here are some startling facts and stats* that might help motivate you to follow the urgent call to eat less and move more.

- 120 million adult Americans, 64.5% of the population, are overweight. That's up from an already whopping 61% in 1999. And it makes us the fattest nation in the world.
- Two out of every three adult Americans are overweight; one in three (31%, 59 million people) are obese.
- The average American adult is gaining 1 to 3 pounds a year.
- Obesity rates among U.S. adults increased 60% in ten years (1990-2000).
- 16% of American adolescents (9 million) aged 12-19 and 15% of children aged 6-11 years are now ove weight. In 1999, 13% of kids aged 6-11 years and 14% of those aged 12-19 years were overweight.
- Since 1980, the percentage of overweight children has nearly doubled; in adolescents, it has nearly tripled.

>>tip

You can ■ stop gaining weight and improve your health simply by taking 2,000 more steps and eating 100 fewer calories each day.

- 60% of American adults do not get enough physical activity (the Surgeon General's recommended 30 minutes per day). 40% get no "leisure" exercise.

- 25% of American adults are sedentary. That increases to 30% for the over 44 crowd, to 35% for people aged 65-75, and to 50% for women 75 and over.

- Lifestyle—specifically, eating too much and moving too little—is the single greatest cause of weight gain in the United States, surpassing age, body type, disease, genetics, side effects of medications (such as steroids), and other factors.

- Approximately 112,000 U.S. deaths a year are associated with being overweight or obese—dwarfing the death rates of accidents, crimes, infectious diseases (flu, pneumonia), and many other diseases.

- The health problems directly linked to overweight and obesity include heart disease, hypertension (high blood pressure), stroke, adult-onset (type 2) diabetes, arthritis, asthma, depression, gall bladder disease, liver disease, and more.

- A weight gain of 11-18 pounds increases the risk of heart disease by 25%. More than 25 pounds puts you in the danger zone—skyrocketing the risk to 200-300%!

• Type 2 diabetes, a debilitating and life threatening consequence of obesity, almost doubled from 1990-2000. It rose 70% in people aged 30-39.

• In 1990, type 2 diabetes was virtually unheard of in children Today, type 2 diabetes, a direct result of obesity, accounts for 50% of new pediatric cases of diabetes. The health problems associated with diabetes include vision loss, high blood pressure, circulatory problems, mood disorders, and increased risk of heart attack, stroke, and early death.

The good news: study after study has shown that virtually everyone—regardless of their age, gender, body type, DNA, weight, and fitness level—can better manage their weight and improve their health by making small, incremental changes in their lifestyles—specifically, in their daily dietary and exercise habits.

Good to Go … Walking, That Is!

Walking is one of the best ways to get the physical activity everybody needs. It can be done virtually anywhere, any time, and at any pace. It doesn't require fancy equipment or specialized training. It can be done alone or with friends. It works all your muscles, not just your legs. Most important, it works!

Walking regularly:

• Significantly reduces the risk of heart disease, stroke, diabetes,

FitnessFACT

The Difference 6K Makes

A lower death rate has been shown in men who take as few as 6,000 steps a day.

hypertension (high blood pressure), arthritis, osteoporosis, and some forms of cancer.

- Strengthens bones, joints, muscles, and tendons, which not only promotes long-term muscular and skeletal health but also reduces the risk of injury during physical activity and as a person ages.
- Reduces "bad" cholesterol (LDL) and raises "good" cholesterol (HDL).
- Helps to lower and prevent high blood pressure.
- Reduces belly and upper-body fat.
- Slows the aging process and increases both physical energy and stamina.
- Strengthens stomach and back muscles, preventing and reducing pot-belly and backaches.
- Is the safest and most effective exercise for pregnant women and seniors (age 55 and older).

The Commitment to Balance Your Energy

The 10,000-Steps-A-Day Program gives you the tools and tips you need to add steps to your day and cut calories from your diet... as easily, seamlessly, and painlessly as chewing gum. It's not about going from 900 to 10,000 steps in one day flat, or in one week,

FitnessFACT
The Pink Ribbon for Walking

Walking is associated with a decreased risk of breast cancer in postmenopausal women, according to a study of overweight but otherwise healthy women aged 21-45. The longest duration of physical activity, which consisted primarily of walking, gave the most benefit but did not need to be vigorous to reduce breast-cancer risk. The cardio-respiratory (heart/lung) fitness of all the study participants improved, and each lost 13-20 pounds and kept it off for a year.

one month, one year, or any prescribed amount of time. It's not about taking 10,000 steps every day or even 10,000 steps any day. It's about tailoring the 10,000-steps-a-day fitness strategy to your body, your personal goals, and your lifestyle. It's about helping you to make healthier activity and eating habits a normal, enjoyable, and comfortable part of your everyday life. Ultimately, it's about helping you to better balance the amount of energy you consume with the amount of energy you expend.

The key word here is "balance." The main reason 120 million adult Americans, 64.5% of the population, and 15% of our kids, are overweight is because they eat too much and move too little. This is what the current U.S. Surgeon General Richard Carmone calls an "energy imbalance," and it cannot be corrected by diet alone. To get fit and stay healthy, you also need to move that body ... and not just once in a while or until you've reached a certain weight or size or shape, but consistently, every day, as a way of life.

The 10,000-Steps-A-Day Program is a low-tech, low-impact, low-cost, and highly effective way to balance your physical output with your food

Bonus Benefits

Walking not only improves your health, it also helps you look and feel better. Walking helps you to:

1. Curb your appetite
2. Melt fat
3. Firm and shape muscles
4. Boost your energy
5. Build your physical stamina
6. Prevent and decrease anxiety and depression
7. Reduce stress
8. Sleep better
9. Enhance your sex drive
10. Relax and enjoy life more

intake. It gives you all the tools and tips you'll need to make health-building exercise and eating a regular and pleasant part of your everyday life—so that you'll actually do it, enjoy it, and get lasting positive results from it.

It is said that a journey of a thousand miles begins with the first step. You've already taken your first step on your journey toward optimal weight and better health, by choosing the 10,000-Steps-A-Day Program as your guide. Now, it's time to find out how to take the next steps toward your ultimate destination—a slimmer, healthier, and happier you.

CHAPTER TWO

ON YOUR MARK
Finding Your Start Point

Walking might be as simple as chewing gum, but walking for fitness—to manage or lose weight and to sustain or improve health—is a little more involved. True, it requires no fancy equipment or special clothing. No fitness center or personal trainer. No membership dues or expiration date. No waiting in line to use the sweat-covered machines. No competition or complicated choreographed routines. But fitness walking is exercise, and the 10,000-Steps-A-Day Program is an exercise program that, while simple, requires conscious effort.

In other words, we can show you the way, but only you can follow through. And your best assurance of achieving your fitness goals is to make new and improved exercise and eating habits a part of your every day life … as routine as brushing your teeth, doing your daily chores, and tucking in your kids at night.

The basic objective of the 10,000-Steps-A-Day Program is to help you balance the energy you exert with the energy you consume, by reducing your daily calories and increasing your daily physical activity—gradually and incrementally, a few calories and a few steps at a time, one day at a

" *Walking is the biggest bang for our buck. Thirty minutes a day of walking will prevent many cases of diabetes, hypertension, and other chronic diseases. Walking is the simplest, easiest way [to exercise] for most people.* **"**

–*Richard Carmone, U.S. Surgeon General*

time. As long as you do that, you will get positive results—inside, where you'll feel them, as well as outside, where you'll see them—whether or not you ever reach 10,000 steps a day. The one sure thing about exercise is that doing something is better than doing nothing. And cutting just 100 calories (10 potato chips) and adding 30 minutes of exercise (about 2000 steps) a day is enough to keep most people from gaining additional weight, and it's "doable" for virtually anybody. All it takes is conscious effort—making the commitment and time to do it. That's where the 10,000-Steps-A-Day Program gives you the advantage.

Studies show that the most effective exercise programs—the ones people stick with and get the best and lasting results from—include specific goals and a way of tracking progress toward those goals. As the saying goes, when you know better, you do better. The 10,000-Steps-A-Day Program gives you the information and tools you need to both set and reach your personal goals.

It all starts with the Step-Counter, the handy gadget included with this book. First, we show you how to use the Step-Counter to determine the average number of steps you currently take in the normal course of your daily life—your "baseline." Next, we help you to determine how many steps you need and want to add, in what increments and at what intervals (over time), based on your body type, age, health, fitness level, lifestyle, and personal goals. Then, we show you how to use the Step-Counter, along with the Daily Step Log, to keep track of your daily steps as you move toward your goal.

Studies indicate that it takes 6 months of doing something repeatedly before the behavior "sets in" and becomes a pattern. Studies also indicate that it usually takes 12 weeks before the results of a new moderate exercise program are measurable, though you will see increases in strength and endurance. That's why the 10,000-Steps-A-Day Program follows a six-month course, which we've broken into two levels to make it even easier: (1) a 90-day plan that advances you toward your daily "stabilizing" goal (adding at least 2,000 steps to your current baseline); (2) a 90-day plan that advances you toward your daily "optimal" goal (up to a total of 10,000 steps per day).

Later, if you're overweight or obese and want to trim additional pounds and inches, we show you how to step it up a notch with the 10,000-Plus Level. Finally, for that finishing touch, we walk you through a basic set of strength training and body sculpting

Simple Science

Calories Consumed > Calories Used = Weight Gain

Calories Consumed = Calories Used = Weight Stability

Calories Consumed < Calories Used = Weight Loss

exercises that you can do at home with little or no equipment.

But first, before you can decide where you're going and how to get there, you need to find out where you are. With your Step-Counter, that's no sweat at all.

Ten Sure Steps to Exercise Success

Pick up virtually any fitness magazine or book, and you'll probably find some words of wisdom or warning about why exercise programs fail. It usually goes something like this: lack of … time, enjoyment, motivation, realistic goals, regularity, variety, support, proper instruction, good eating habits, rewards, etc. Although all those lack-ofs certainly can and often do derail an exercise program, I've found it is much more encouraging, empowering, and effective to focus on why exercise programs succeed.

People who get beneficial and lasting results from exercise tend to:

1. Make the commitment. Identifying why you want to exercise will help you to commit your time and effort toward reaching your personal fitness objective.

2. Set realistic and specific goals. Knowing your current level of fitness (weight, strength, stamina, health issues, etc.) and the level of

fitness you wish to achieve and sustain are the first two steps toward figuring out how and how quickly to move safely and steadily toward your goals.

3. Keep an exercise log. Recording your daily exercise activities and tracking the results not only enables you to monitor your progress and identify necessary changes, it is also a great motivator. Seeing that you're taking more steps and with greater ease—even when you aren't seeing a significant change in weight, size, or cholesterol levels—will encourage you to at least stick with it, if not add more exercise and/or decrease calories.

4. Start small and build slowly. Fitting your exercise routine to your current level of fitness and then gradually increasing the amount and difficulty of exercise as your body strengthens ensures against discomfort, frustration, and injury—and, ultimately, keeps you moving. So, if you lean toward all-or-nothing exercise thinking or quick-fix fitness strategies, ditch them now; they never work.

5. Do a variety of activities you enjoy. Engaging in physical activities you genuinely enjoy and adding interesting new activities or doing a favorite activity a new way now and then will prevent boredom and keep you motivated and moving.

6. Have good information and instruction. When you know better, you do better. Knowing how to exercise properly and knowing the beneficial effects of proper exercise as well as the ill effects of inade-

quate and improper exercise go a long way toward getting and keeping you on the right fitness track for you.

7. Allow and plan for "off" days. Stuff happens. You get sick; you get distracted; you get injured; you get busy; you get tired; you get bored; you travel; you get the blues. Other things take priority: children, holidays, family, work, friendships. And sometimes you just can't fit in exercise or just don't feel like it. Acknowledging and preparing for those inevitable slips and slides with contingency and get-back-in-the-saddle plans will help prevent major set-backs and withdrawals.

8. Get sufficient hydration and proper nutrition. Eating the right foods in the right amounts and drinking enough water not only gives your body the energy it needs to operate efficiently, helping both to improve health and manage weight, it also gives you the energy you need to exercise, helping to ensure against overexertion and dehydration.

9. Get sufficient rest and relaxation. Getting enough down time increases both the effectiveness of and your enjoyment of exercise while decreasing the risk of injury and of you quitting because you're feeling overloaded or overtired.

10. Reward progress. Giving yourself a tangible reward when you reach each goal along the way provides an added incentive for moving forward. Rewards are especially effective when you reach

FitnessFACT

Tally Ho!

As reported in the esteemed journal Preventative Medicine, in an experiment dubbed the "Prince Edward Island First-Step Program" (Canada), 106 subjects wore step counters before and during a twelve-week walking program in which they were tasked with increasing their daily steps. Before the experiment the subjects averaged 7,000 steps a day; while wearing the step counters, they averaged 10,500 steps a day. By the end of the program, the participants also had achieved a significant decrease in weight, waist size, and resting heart rate.

a plateau and the good results going on inside might not be immediately obvious on the outside. For most people, it is best to stick with rewards other than food—for example, a facial, or a new outfit, or a night on the town, or for those big milestones, a vacation (preferably a walking tour).

Meet Your Step-Counter: The Ideal Walking Partner

Take a look at the small device that came with this book. It doesn't look like much, does it? Well, don't let looks deceive you; the Step-Counter is one of the powerful fitness tools you'll ever meet. The strength of the Step-Counter lies in its accountability. It takes the guesswork out of estimating your daily activity, spelling it out in black and white. A number of factors—feeling tired or stressed, being overly busy or sick, the weather or the time of year—can affect your perception of how active you've been on a given day, causing you to overestimate or underestimate how much you've

Easy as 1-2-3

One of the beauties of your Step-Counter is that it is so easy to use. Just:

1. Set the Step-Counter to zero (0) by pressing the Reset button.
2. Clip the Step-Counter to your belt, waistband, or pocket, directly above the knee (about 6 or 7 inches left or right of your belly button). Make sure it is secure, right side up, and horizontal to the ground (not on an angle or dangling).
3. Start walking.

exercised. Incredibly, just knowing how many steps you've taken—confirming that you're making progress or alerting you that you're slipping up—can motivate you to continue the momentum or to exercise more.

A step counter is simply a pedometer that counts the number of steps you take by sensing the motion your body makes when you walk (or jog, climb stairs, work out on a treadmill, do leg lifts, etc.). Step counters can be set to count the number of steps you take during a specific activity (a walk in the park, for example), a specific distance (one mile), a specific interval of time (30 minutes), or an entire day. For busy people, it is an ideal way to chalk up (and encourage you to increase) the "lifestyle" steps you take outside of any formal exercise routine—when cleaning house, running errands, walking to the copy machine or to speak with a coworker, climbing stairs, coaching your child's soccer team, etc.

Step counters have been around for years. The older models, however, sometimes received poor marks for being clunky and inaccurate. Technology has vastly improved the size, shape, weight, and functionality of step counters, and highly accurate digital electronics has replaced the less accurate mechanical balls and levers of early models. Recent studies of several different brands of step counters have shown that at normal walking speeds, electronic models were 97% accurate, far surpassing the abilities of the mechanical models. At faster speeds, the digital step counters were even more accurate (up to 99%), although they were slightly less precise at very slow speeds, such as the walking pace of an elderly person.

Your 10,000 Steps Step-Counter is a compact, lightweight, digital model that has been trial-tested for accuracy at normal and fast walking speeds. It is comfortable to wear and slim enough that it doesn't jut out unattractively and obtrusively. The manufacturers recommend wearing it on your waistband, six inches to the left or right of your bellybutton. However, studies have shown that digital step counters are equally accurate no matter where on your waistline you wear them. Experts have also found that accuracy is the same for both obese and normal-weight walkers, and that accuracy is not adversely affected by the length or speed of your stride.

Your goal is to find your baseline and then to gradually increase that number over the next six months, working toward the optimal 10,000 steps a day. Wearing your Step-Counter every day will help you to do that.

>>tip

As an ■ extra precaution against losing or breaking your Step-Counter or inadvertently bumping (and pressing) a button, slip a shoestring through the clip and tie or pin the string to your waistband, belt loop, or pocket. Although the clip usually holds the Step-Counter securely in place, bending (for example, to tie your shoe or to sit down), walking briskly or on a rough surface, or moving abruptly could jar it loose.

To Determine Your Steps per Mile

Your Step-Counter cannot automatically calculate miles as you walk. However, it is fairly easy to calculate your distance in miles once you know how many steps you take in a mile.

1. Find a measured mile (for example, the distance between two green mileage markers on a road).

2. Reset your Step-Counter to zero and attach it to your waistband or belt.

3. Walk the measured mile.

4. Record your steps-per-mile in the front of your Daily Step Log.

Another simple way to determine your steps-per-mile is to walk one lap on a high-school or college track, wearing your Step-Counter. Each lap is exactly a quarter-mile. After completing one lap, multiply the number of steps on your Step-Counter by four, and you will have the number of steps you take in a mile.

To track your miles walked: If you want to track the number of miles you take daily or during a specific walking session:

1. Walk with your Step-Counter activated.

2. Record the number of steps taken in your Daily Step Log.

3. Divide the total number of steps taken by your steps-per-mile number.

Finding Your Baseline

Now that you're familiar with your Step-Counter, you're probably anxious to put it into action and start walking. As long as you have no physical limitations or health issues that might prevent you from "just doing it," as the Nike slogan goes, there is no reason why you couldn't put on your walking shoes, clip on your Step-Counter, and get moving right now. And if you want to do that, go ahead and give it a whirl.

But getting the most out of the 10,000-Steps-A-Day Program involves customizing the exercise program to fit your body, lifestyle, and goals. And that begins with determining your step baseline—the number of steps you currently take, on average, during a normal day, which may or may not include formal exercise. To find your step baseline:

• Wear your Step-Counter all day every day for two weeks (14 days) while going about your life-as usual.

• Every morning, make sure your Step-Counter is set to zero (if it is not, press Reset), clip it to your belt or waistband, and wear it continuously throughout the day,

>>tip

Give Your Step-Counter a Trial Run

To test your Step-Counter: set it to zero (press Reset), clip it to your waistband or belt, and take 50 steps at a normal pace, counting the steps yourself as you walk. Check the number of steps recorded on your Step-Counter. If the reading is not within 5 steps, plus or minus, of your actual steps—that is, if it counted fewer than 45 steps or more than 55 steps—reposition the Step-Counter and try again. Repositioning the Step-Counter usually resolves any discrepancy, though it might take a few tries.

including during any exercise activity and while relaxing. Don't do anything to change your normal routine.

• At bedtime, remove the Step-Counter, write the number of steps you took that day in your Daily Step Log, and press the Reset button.

• At the end of one week (or two weeks, if you opt for the more accurate two-week baseline), use a calculator to add together the number of daily steps you took for the week (or two weeks) and then divide that sum by 7 (or by 14). Round up (or down) to the nearest whole number. This is your baseline—your average daily number of steps.

For the sake of simplicity, the daily entries in the sample baseline log, above, are all simple, even numbers. In reality, the number of steps a person takes on any given day is more likely to be 3,527 steps rather than a tidy 3,500. Every step counts, so make sure to record the actual number of steps displayed on your Step-Counter in your log each day.

You'll also probably notice that the number of steps you take varies from day to day. For example, it could be as few as 900 steps some days and as many as 2,500 on other days. That is not unusual, and you should not modify your usual physical activity during the 14-day baseline period. In order to set an attainable goal and to create a program that will be the most effective for you, you must first determine an accurate (and real) baseline, which is impossible to do if you modify your normal routine to add or even out your daily steps during the baseline period.

Once you've established your baseline—and, if you have any physical limitations or health issues, checked with your doctor— you're ready to move on to the next steps in the 10,000-Steps-A-DayProgram: setting your personal step goals.

When to Check with Your Doctor

If in doubt, it's best to ask. Even if you are fit as a fiddle and already exercise regularly, it's smart to check with your doctor before starting a new exercise or significantly increasing your physical activity. And anyone with compromised health and/or physical disabilities should always check with her or his doctor before starting any new physical activity, including one as simple and easy as walking. That does not necessarily mean that people with impaired health or physical limitations are unable to participate in the program; in fact, walking is perfectly safe for and is known to help improve many serious conditions. However, the person might need to tailor the program to his or her specific needs—based on their doctor's advice and with the doctor's full consent.

Before you begin your 10,000-Steps-A-Day Program, please take a few minutes to answer the following yes-or-no questions:

>>**tip**

Do not ■ wear your Step-Counter while submersed in water. Take it off while bathing, showering, swimming, or engaging in other water sports.

• Has your doctor ever told you that you have or are at high risk of developing heart problems, high blood pressure, or diabetes?
• Have you ever had a heart attack or a stroke?
• Has anyone in your family had a heart attack or a stroke or died of cardiovascular disease before the age of 50?
• Do you ever experience pains or extreme pressure in your chest or on the left side of your neck, your left shoulder, or your left arm when you are physically active?
• Do you often feel breathless, dizzy, faint, and/or ligh headed during or immediately after physical activity?
• Do you have bone, joint, or tendon problems, such as arthritis, osteoporosis, chin splints, knee tendonitis, sprained ankle, sciatica,

FitnessFACT
City Striders

When it comes to exercise, the wholesomeness of small-town living versus the evils of big-city living may be more myth than fact. As reported in Medicine & Science in Sports & Exercise magazine, nationwide study of leisure-time and exercise found that people in large cities had the highest rates of daily activity, while rural residents (especially in the South) had the highest prevalence of inactivity and lowest levels of physical fitness. Score one for the concrete jungle.

pulled Achilles tendon?, etc.

- Are you a man over age 40 or a woman over age 50 who has not had a physical exam within the past two years?
- Have you been sedentary (little or no physical activity) for more than 6 months?
- Do you smoke or have asthma, allergies, emphysema, or any other lung condition?
- Do you have any chronic disorders, such as multiple sclerosis, lupus, chronic fatigue syndrome, fibromyalgia, etc.?
- Do you have residual pain or persistent symptoms from a previous injury to your muscular or skeletal systems?
- Do you currently have pain, weakness, and/or swelling of any joint, tendon, muscle, or bone?
- Do you take medication to treat or control any chronic medical condition, including high blood pressure, high cholesterol, diabetes, etc.?
- Do you abuse alcohol or other drugs?
- Are you pregnant?

Sample Step Log Baseline Entry

	Mon.	Tue.	Wed.	Thu.	Fri.	Sat.	Sun.
Week 1	3,500	5,300	4,200	5,000	3,600	5,800	3,600
Week 2	3,800	6,100	3,200	4,700	4,300	5,200	3,700
Totals	7,300	11,400	7,400	9,700	7,900	11,000	7,300

Number of Steps Taken During Trial: 62,000 (sum of daily totals for both weeks)
Baseline: 62,000 (number of steps) ÷ 14 (days) = 4,429 (average daily steps)

- Do you have a health problem or physical condition not mentioned here that might give you pause to start a new physical activity?

If you answered "yes" to any of these questions, consult with your doctor before beginning this or any exercise program. In most cases, the doctor will approve walking as an exercise and will recommend any necessary limitations, modifications, precautions, and special equipment or treatments (such as a knee brace or taking an aspirin).

CHAPTER THREE

GET SET

Custom-fit Your Step Program to Your Body, Life, and Goals

A recent study by the President's Council of Physical Fitness and Sports concluded that setting realistic goals and using a step counter to monitor daily steps is the dynamic duo when it comes to motivating people to exercise regularly to reach their exercise-related goals. The goal of the 10,000-Steps-A-Day Program is to help you add 30 minutes of physical activity to your day. According to the U.S. Surgeon General, that is enough physical activity to manage your weight, reduce your risk of chronic diseases, and help you lead a longer, healthier life—a conclusion backed by numerous scientific studies.

Another important goal of the 10,000-Steps-A-Day Program is to help you fit walking (or an equivalent physical activity) into your everyday life. Why? Because making physical activity a habit—as second-nature as brushing your teeth or doing the dishes—plays a huge role in achieving your fitness goals.

Now that you know your baseline (the average number of steps you currently take each day), it is time to determine how many steps you need to add each day to achieve your own fitness goals and how best to add them. And that hinges on your answer to the most important question of all: why?

Identify Your Why

It is virtually impossible to commit to something if you aren't clear why you're doing it in the first place. To devote the time and effort it takes to succeed at anything, particularly something new and the least bit out of your comfort zone, there has to be a good reason (or reasons) behind it. And you must be honest, realistic, and specific in identifying those reasons. To say that you're starting a new exercise program because you want to "lose weight" or "get fit" or "be healthier" or "live longer" is well and fine. Those are all sound reasons, and chances are, 99% of the people asked would give similar rationale for starting a new exercise activity. But those rather reasons alone are usually not personal and specific enough to motivate you to make the necessary changes, both within yourself and in your daily life, to stick with the exercise.

For most people, it is much easier to find reasons not to start or continue an exercise program than it is to get real about their personal reasons for doing it—and that is why so many people are inconsistent with and then quit an exercise activity. Doing some soul-searching upfront to get to the bottom of precisely why you

> **"We are under-exercised as a nation. We look, instead of play. We ride, instead of walk. Our existence deprives us of the minimum of physical activity essential for healthy living. "**
>
> *–John F. Kennedy*

want to trim down, tone up, or improve your health will help you to: (1) set attainable and meaningful goals, (2) choose physical activities that fit your interests and lifestyle, (3) motivate you to exercise consistently, (4) better enjoy the activity itself; (5) appreciate the small gains along the way; and, (6) ultimately, reach your goals.

Operation Motivation Questionnaire

Ready to identify your why? Just grab a pen or pencil and some blank paper (or write your answers in the book), and answer these simple but revealing questions. If more than one multiple-choice answer applies, either check all that apply or number your responses in order of their importance to you. Skip any question that does not apply. When you're done filling out the questionnaire, go back and review your responses and then keep them in mind when you set your goals for your *10,000-Steps-A-Day Program.*

1. I want to increase (or change) my physical activity primarily because:

    ___ My doctor recommended it

    ___ My spouse or other loved one(s) asked me to

____ I believe it is something I need to do

____ It is something I want to do

2. How satisfied are you with your current level of physical fitness, on a scale of 1-10? ____

3. How satisfied are you with the way you look, on a scale of 1-10? ____

4. How satisfied are you with the way you feel, on a scale of 1-10? ____

5. How concerned are you about your health or level of fitness, on a scale of 0-10? ____

6. What are your specific health and/or fitness concerns? That my physical condition does or might:

____ Interfere with my ability to meet my responsibilities (job, home, family)

____ Limit my lifestyle options

____ Prevent me from doing the things I like and want to do

____ Have an adverse affect on the way people perceive me

____ Diminish my quality of life

____ Cause chronic illness

____ Shorten my life

____ Other (specify)

What are the three things you like best about yourself?

_____

_____

_____

Name the one thing you want most to change about yourself:

_____

_____

_____

What are the three things you like best about your life?

_____

_____

_____

Name the one thing you want most to change about your life:

_____

_____

_____

Name the three most important ways in which being more fit (or sustaining your fitness) might enhance your life: (For example, "Enable me to keep up with and enjoy more physical activities with my children," "Feel more attractive and confidant," and "Continue gardening and playing tennis through my middle and senior years.")

_____

_____

_____

What are your greatest barrier(s) to exercising regularly? (Remember to number in order of importance in your life.)

_____ Lack of time

_____ Lack of resources (exercise equipment, place to exercise, can't afford gym or trainer)

_____ Lack of support from spouse, family, friends, employer

_____ Lack of motivation

_____ Lack of belief that I can achieve my desired level of fitness

_____ Other: _____

_____

For each of the top three barriers that prevent you from exercising regularly, name one change you can make in your life to reduce or remove that barrier. (Feel free to answer for all barriers that apply.):

1._____

_____

_____

2._____

_____

_____

3._____

_____

_____

It's About Time

Twenty-five percent of people who start a new exercise program quit within the first week; another 25% quit within the first six months. What is the most frequently cited reason for quitting? Lack of time—not being able to fit an "extra" 60, 45, 30, or even 10 minutes of exercise into their already jam-packed lives.

In a perfect world, we would all do 60 minutes of cardiovascular exercise every morning. Later that day, after a few, small healthy meals and plenty of water, we would lift weights for 30 minutes. In the late afternoon, after our children have come home from school, where they've already had 60 minutes of physical education, we would spend an hour before dinner with them, kicking a soccer ball, shooting hoops, skipping rope, or jumping on the trampoline. Later in the evening, after a balanced dinner complete with two servings of vegetables, you and your spouse would do 20 minutes of stretching and calisthenics or yoga to help melt away stress and tension and improve flexibility.

Does this sound like Fantasyland? Of course it does. Most Americans work like mules to afford the basic necessities and a few simple luxuries for their families. As each year goes by, we work longer hours both in our jobs and at home, sacrificing time we would spend with our family and on our own mental and physical health. The United States tops the worldwide list of hours worked per week; meanwhile, as a nation, we have become chronically sleep-deprived.

So, when the Surgeon General recommends 30 minutes a day of physical activity—on top of all the running around we do in the course of our daily lives—it begs the question: Where do we get that extra 30 minutes a day? More to the point, how are you going to fit 30 minutes of walking into your busy life?

The short answer is: by adding steps to "life" activities you already do—in increments of a few extra steps and 3, 5, 8 minutes of your time. And by adding new or scheduling more time for exercise activities you like to do—in intervals of 10, 20, and eventually 30 minutes at a time. When you start adding steps here and there, you'll be surprised at how quickly they add up, at how many more calories you'll burn, and at how much better you'll look and feel.

And isn't it time you took that step toward better health?

FitnessFACT

Slay Your Inner Naysayer

Your Fitness Profile

When starting a new exercise routine, most people work out too hard too soon, which leads to discomfort, injuries, frustration, and burn out. It doesn't take long before they get discouraged and quit. Getting real about your current level of fitness, establishing a reasonable starting point, and increasing your physical activity gradually, in sensible intervals, will help you to avoid that kind of no-win situation.

For the majority of people, the number-one barrier to exercising regularly is their own negative self-talk, telling them they don't really need to exercise and/or that it won't work for them. Here's a reality check: Everyone benefits from exercise; studies show that even elderly people using walkers benefit from that activity. And exercising regularly always works if you do it enough, do it right, and do it over the long-term.

The lovely and late actress Jeanne Moreau once said, "We have so many words for states of mind and so few words for the state of the body." That still holds true. Most people think of fitness and exercise in all-or-nothing terms. They think of themselves as either fit or not fit, with no intermediate levels of fitness in between, and if they put themselves in the "not fit" category, all too often they then tell themselves that getting fit is "mission next-to impossible." Too many people have the mistaken notion that if they don't exercise long and hard, like top athletes in competitive training, they might as well not exercise at all. In reality,

>>tip

Walking normally, you take about 70 steps a minute.

very few people have the ability, time, or desire to do formal, strenuous work-outs several hours a day—and it isn't necessary to attaining and managing your optimal weight and to improving and sustaining your health.

"Getting real" about your physical condition means taking stock of both the physical state of your body and the fitness state of your mind. If you're a couch potato, admit you're a couch potato—so that you can then figure out why you're a couch potato (which, assuredly, has to do with your attitude and personal interests as well as your physical condition) and what you can do, and are likely to do, to get off the couch and moving, a little more each day.

Sure, the 10,000-Steps-A-Day program is, at its core, about walking … and walking is simple and easy. In fact, you can start walking right now and do it almost any time and anywhere, without any preliminary evaluating or planning or training—as long as you don't overdo it. If you're ready to walk, go for a walk—now, today. But don't sabotage the effectiveness of your new exercise program by neglecting to zero in on where you are on the fitness scale now.

Size Matters

Knowing your current weight and body fat content as well as your "ideal" weight and body fat content will help you to set realistic exercise goals and to custom-fit your 10,000-Steps-A-Day Program to meet those goals.

When it comes to your health, being too fat or too thin does matter. Being 20% overweight doubles the risk of hypercholesterolemia (a serum cholesterol level exceeding 250 mg/dl), triples the risk of diabetes and high blood pressure, and increases the risk of heart disease by 60%. By the same token, being severely underweight increases the risk of injury and chronic conditions, including bone and joint disorders. To enable your body to store energy and to cool itself properly and to ensure a body composition that sufficiently supports (muscle) and cushions (fat) organs and bones, most health experts recommend a body fat percentage of about 24% for women and 15% for men.

Exercise physiologists typically recommend that people stay within 5% of the optimal weight for their individual height and frame, also known as "body mass index" (BMI). The BMI is not a precise, one-size-fits-all gauge, however. For example, the weight of a muscular athlete with little body fat may well exceed the BMI for his or her height, yet that heavier weight will be perfectly "normal" and pose no serious health risks for that person (assuming he or she has no underlying health problems). By the same token, an inactive thin person may fall within his or her BMI but actually have too little muscle and even too much fat, which weakens bones, joints, and

FitnessFACT

Time Crunch or Time Out?

According to one study, the leisure time of working adult Americans has dropped from 26 to 17 hours per week since 1970. Not so, says the Harris Poll, which reports that American adults have averaged 19-20 hours a week of leisure time every year since 1989. According to the U.S. Bureau of Labor Statistics' "American Time Use Study," which surveyed 21,000 people aged 15 and over in 2003—most adults have, on average, 5.1 hours a day of "free" time. Yet, only one-third spend 30 minutes of that time exercising. Instead, the majority use 50% of their free time watching TV. The second most-favorite American pastime? Reading, another sedentary activity. As the saying goes, old couch-potato habits die hard. All the more reason to use a fitness program that helps you replace unhealthy habits with a healthy one you can fit smoothly into your life: walking.

muscles and reduces energy and stamina.

Body composition (the ratio of muscle versus fat in your body) and body type (how fat is distributed in your body) are often better indicators of health risk and fitness level than BMI.

You've no doubt heard of the three most commonly recognized body types: endomorph (curvy), ectomorph (willowy), and mesomorph (muscular).

Endomorphs, who are often pear-shaped, tend to have a high capacity for fat storage and are susceptible to weight gain and obesity, which increases their risk of diabetes, high blood pressure, stroke, some cancers, and heart disease. According to the American Heart Association, people who tend to collect fat in their upper bodies (back, chest, stomach, arms), as is the tendency with some endomorphs, are at significantly higher risk of heart disease. When coupled with high triglyceride (bad cholesterol) levels, the risk is even higher.

Also at higher risk of cardiovascular disease are overweight mesomorphs. Fortunately for mesomorphs, they tend to burn off fat with exercise relatively easily.

Ectomorphs, who tend to be thin and to have small bones and muscles, but can be of any height, are more prone to bone and joint disorders, such as arthritis and osteoporosis. Having too little muscle and either too little or too much fat can put excessive stress on the typically delicate ecotomorphic frame.

Other factors—some within your control but many outside of your control—play a role in determining your optimal weight and shape and in determining how quickly and easily you can achieve it. Genetics, for example, can inhibit or accelerate the rate at which and the extent to which you can lose weight and shape up. All diet and exercise things being equal, some people just shed pounds, drop fat, and build muscle faster. Certain medical conditions (such as thyroid disorders) and environmental factors (such as stress) can affect your metabolism (the rate and efficiency with which your body burns calories), muscle mass and strength, and how and where your body stores and burns fat. Genetics can limit or enhance the speed and extent to which you respond to exercise and positive dietary changes. Age and gender also factor in. Generally, men have a higher metabolism and lower fat-to-muscle ratio than women.

Nevertheless, someone who leans toward the endomorphic side needs to understand that he or she may never be able to reach their super-lean goal of 8% or 12% body fat and still maintain good health. In fact, they are likely to look and feel great at twice that rate. Similarly, someone with mostly ectomorphic characteristics may never achieve 21-inch biceps he or she desires. And someone with the muscular and sometimes square build of a mesomorph may never achieve the cone, hourglass, or long willowy shape of their dreams.

Bottom line: every body is different. Knowing your body's unique characteristics will help you to better assess your fitness potential and to arrive at goals that are both realistic and achievable.

Whatever your body type and physical make-up, the evidence is clear: being overweight, out of shape, or overly fat is hazardous to your health. The evidence is equally clear that walking is an ideal exercise for any body size, shape, or type. It burns fat, builds muscle, strengthens bones, and smoothes out lumps and bumps. And virtually any body can do it. What varies somewhat from one person to another in determining individual exercise efficiency are: how you walk, how much you walk, and the exercise you do in addition to walking (such as strength training and stretching) to get the results you want for your body type.

Body Type Quiz

Most people are predominately one of the three classic body types—ectomorph, endomorph, or mesomorph. But no one is 100% one type or another, and all people have characteristics of one or both of the other two types. This short quiz will give you a general idea of your body type.

1. You tend to be leaner in:
   a. Your lower body
   b. Your upper body or mid-section
   c. Your entire body

2. You tend to carry more weight in:
   a. Your upper body (back, chest, stomach, arms)
   b. Your lower body (hips, thighs, buttocks) or both your upper and lower body
   c. Your stomach and buttocks, if at all

3. The most difficult part of your body to slim down is:
   a. Your upper body
   b. Your lower body or both your upper and lower
   c. Not very difficult or no need to trim down

FitnessFACT
Too Far Gone to Get Back On Track?

Don't believe it! In fact, if you have been inactive for a while and start exercising, you will experience improvements even more rapidly than people who have a history of being active.

4. Your shape most resembles a:

   a. Pear, apple, or hourglass

   b. Ruler

   c. Cone (inverted pyramid)

5. Your frame (bone size) is:

   a. Small to medium

   b. Medium to large

   c. Small (regardless of height)

If you answered (a) at least twice, your body type is primarily endomorphic.

If you answered (b) at least twice, your body type is primarily mesomorphic.

If you answered (c) at least twice, your body type is ectomorphic.

Body Composition

Although your fat-to-muscle ratio is a better indicator of your fitness level than your weight-to-height ratio or your weight alone, it is not the end-all. Like BMI, the guidelines for body composition do not factor in genetics, medical conditions, and certain other factors that affect your weight as it relates to your fitness level, but it does factor in age and gender as well as height and weight. Unlike BMI, there is no universal set of standards for body composition. Consequently, the body composition reference points cited by various fitness experts and publications can vary greatly, and many are not based on scientific research.

Although there are benefits to knowing your body fat percentage, it is not imperative to your 10,000-Steps-A-Day Program. Being aware that you have excess body fat and of where it tends to collect in your body is sufficient to set your goals and start walking. If you do want to find out your body composition, you can have your fat percent measured by a practitioner measure or you can do it yourself, using one of these three common methods:
• Underwater (hydrostatic) weighing
• Body fat scales (bioelectrical impedance)
• Skin-fold calipers

Body Composition Standards

The following body fat reference ranges (for adults) were developed by the American College of Sport's Medicine based on extensive scientific research.

FitnessFACT
Goal One: Lose Weight

By a landslide, weight loss is the most common goal of people starting a new exercise activity. Too bad more than 50% stop exercising when they don't get the quick-fix they expect--because if they would just stick with it, study after study has shown that they would slowly but surely shed pounds and inches.

Health Standards: percent of body fat that generally does not increase risk of health problems

Fitness Standards: percent of body fat that generally reduces the risk of health problems

High Risk: percent of body fat that usually poses significant risk of health problems

So ... What's Your BMI?

This is probably not the question you want someone to ask you at a social gathering—unless you're built like Madonna or Matthew McConaughey. But it is one you might want to ask yourself when setting your exercise goals for working toward or sustaining your optimal weight ... and (while you're at it) your ideal body shape.

Below is a partial body mass index (BMI) table; it is for adult men and women. Several government and health organizations post a complete index on their Web sites and some offer the tables in print form as well. There are also dozens of BMI calculators online and on the market, which calculate your BMI to your exact weight.

BMI Formula

The formula for determining BMI, in kilograms and meters, is:

weight in kg ÷ height in m2

To compute your BMI, in pounds (your weight) and inches (your height):

> your weight x 705 ÷ your height ÷ your height again = your BMI

BMI Standards

Underweight	< 18.5
Healthy weight	18.5-24.9
Overweight	25.0-29.9
Obese I	30.0-34.9
Obese II	35.0-39.9
Obese III	40+

Note: The body mass index looks only at weight versus height and does not factor in age, gender, genetics, any medical conditions you might have, any medications you might be taking, or the natural variances in muscle weight and bone weight between people. A healthy weight for you might be higher than the BMI standards. So, think of your BMI as a rough guide. A more accurate indicator of your fitness level and health status is the percentage of fat versus muscle in your body—your "body composition."

Begin at Your Beginning

The goal of the 10,000-Steps-A-Day Program is to help you to be more physically active every day of the week. Sitting around Monday through Saturday and then taking a three-hour strenuous hike on Sunday to try to make up for it is not effective or wise, and is more apt to make you sore than fit. Increasing your daily activity gradually—by incrementally adding steps to your baseline at a pace and in a way that is right for your personal fitness level and goals—is key to making the end goal of being physically active every day a reality.

The following Lifestyle Activity Level Chart, Walking Fitness Test, and Walking Level Chart will help you to find the best starting point for you.

Walking Fitness Level Test

James Rippe, M.D.—cardiologist, director of the Rippe Lifestyle Institute, former medical director of the Rockport Walking Institute, and the guru of "fitness walking—developed this formula to help novice, intermediate, and experienced walkers assess their fitness level by walking a mile on a level, smooth surface. To test your walking fitness level, warm up for 5 minutes by stretching your calves and hamstrings, and then time yourself as you walk a mile as quickly as you can.

Under age 30: Walking a mile in 13 minutes means you're in great shape.

Are You Big-Boned?

For a quick and easy way to gauge your frame size, just measure your wrist.

	Small Frame	Medium Frame	Large Frame
Adult Male	under 6 inches	6-7 inches	over 7 inches
Adult Female	under 5 inches	5-6 inches	over 6 inches

Age 30-39: Walking a mile in 14 minutes means you're in great shape.

Age 40-49: Walking a mile in just under 15 minutes (14 minutes, 42 seconds) puts you at the top level of fitness for your age group.

Age 50-69: Walking a mile in 15 minutes is excellent.

Age 70 or over: Walking a mile in 18 minutes means you're in very good shape for your age.

CAUTION: If you experience any adverse symptoms during the test, slow down or stop. If you are very overweight, obese, or in poor health, do not do this test.

Setting Your Exercise Program Goals

Now that you've got a handle on your physical fitness profile—your reasons for wanting to exercise, your current physical condition, and your baseline (average number of steps you take each day in the normal course of living)—you can set attainable, meaningful, and measurable goals for your 10,000-Steps-A-Day Program. Remember, this is not about rushing to increase your steps to

10,000 a day overnight. It's about increasing your steps gradually, in ways and at a pace that fit your physical condition and lifestyle.

Let's start by looking at the basic guidelines for American adults, as outlined by the U.S. Surgeon General:

- To reduce the risk of chronic disease, you need 30 minutes of moderate intensity (normal) walking a day on top of your normal lifestyle activities.
- To manage your weight (prevent weight gain, sustain weight loss), you need to do about 60 minutes of moderate to brisk walking a day, while ensuring that your caloric intake does not exceed your energy output (calories burned).
- To lose weight, you need to do 60 to 90 minutes of moderate to brisk walking, while ensuring that your caloric intake is less than your energy output.
- To further increase muscle mass, muscle strength, agility, flexibility, and stamina, you need to add strength training and resistance exercises such as calisthenics, Pilates, and yoga two or three times a week—in addition to your daily walking.

Sound overwhelming? Relax. It's really not. And it's much easier when you break it down into smaller pieces. For example, you can start by increasing your steps by 20% over your baseline each week for the first three months of the program. At the end of those 12 weeks, you can review your progress—which you've been recording

	Age	Women	Men
Health Standards	<40 yrs.	20-35%	8-22%
	>40 yrs.	25-38%	10-25%
Fitness Standards	<40 yrs.	16-28%	5-15%
	>40 yrs.	20-33%	7-18%
High Risk			
Obesity	<40 yrs	>35%	>22%
	>40 yrs.	>25%	>25%
Inadequate Fat	any age	<12-14%	<3-5%

in your Daily Step Log—and then reassess your goals and either continue increasing your steps by 20% a week, or slow it down or step it up for the next three-month leg of the program. Your end-goal: after 24 weeks, by the end of the six-month program, you will have made sufficient and regular exercise your habit for life.

Let's say your baseline is 2,500 steps a day and your goal for each of the first 3 weeks is to increase your daily steps by 20%. That's an additional 500 steps a day. Walking at a moderate to brisk clip, you can take 100 steps in one minute; so, adding 500 steps means adding about 5 minutes of walking each day. And anyone can fit 5 more minutes of walking into their day.

Another option is to set your start-up goal at adding a 5-minute, 10-minute, or 15-minute walking session (depending on your level of fitness and personal goals) to each day for, say, the first month. And then increase each walking session by 2 to 5 minutes per week, until you are walking 30 to 45 minutes a day by the end of the first leg (12 weeks) or the final leg (24 weeks) of your program.

Yet another option is to make your first goal the highest number of daily steps you took during your two-week baseline test. Don't choose a higher number, which could put you at risk of injury. Feel free to select a smaller number of steps, but preferably not the least number. Let's say you set your first goal at 3,000 steps, which you reached or exceeded 4 times during your two-week baseline period. After sustaining that goal of walking about 3,000 steps a day for 2 to 4 weeks, review your progress (conveniently recorded in your log) and reevaluate your goals to determine whether you're ready to advance to your next planned step-increase goal or whether you want to adjust it up or down or just continue at 3,000 steps for the next week or two.

A simple option is to set your goals at accumulating a certain number of additional steps (over your baseline) by the end of the first leg of your program (12 weeks) and a certain number of additional steps by the end of the second leg of your program (24 weeks).

Probably the easiest option is break each of the two legs of the

program into 2-week, 3-week, or 4-week intervals and set your
goal at adding 50 to 100 daily steps per interval, until you reach
10,000 steps. You can use different intervals for the first and second legs of the program (for example, breaking weeks 1-12 into
two-week intervals and weeks 13-24 into four-week intervals), but
it is best not to vary the intervals within each three-month leg of
the program.

Which goal-setting method you use and which goals you choose
are completely up to you. Do what you think will work best for
you. If a few weeks into the program you decide that it's not working for you, try to come up with a different goal strategy that does.
And if you don't reach a goal, don't get discouraged. Just do your
best, reassess, and try again.

One of the advantages of the 10,000-Steps-A-Day Program is
that you can set and periodically adjust your goals at whatever
number of steps, in whatever increments, and at whatever intervals you want. The important things are to remain flexible, to be
persistent as you move toward the optimum goal of 10,000 steps a
day, and not to overreach or overdo.

For beginners ("Novice" and "Moderate" levels), in particular,
it is better to increase distance (number of steps) and frequency
than it is to increase duration (amount of time) and intensity. If
you're healthy, trim (not greatly overweight or obese), physically

Body Mass Index Table (partial)

BMI	20	21	22	23	24	25	26	27	28	29	30
Height	**Body Weight (pounds)**										
5'2"	109	115	120	126	131	136	142	147	153	158	164
5'3"	113	118	124	130	135	141	146	152	158	163	169
5'4"	116	122	128	134	140	145	151	157	163	169	174
5'5"	120	126	132	138	144	150	156	162	168	174	180
5'6"	124	130	136	142	148	155	161	167	173	179	186
5'7"	127	134	140	146	153	159	166	172	178	185	191
5'8"	131	138	144	151	158	164	171	177	184	190	197
5'9"	135	142	149	155	162	169	176	182	189	196	203
5'10"	139	146	153	160	167	174	181	188	195	202	209
5'11"	143	150	157	165	172	179	186	193	200	208	215
6'	147	154	162	169	177	184	191	199	206	213	221
6'1"	151	159	166	174	182	189	197	204	212	219	227
6'2"	155	163	171	179	186	194	202	210	218	225	233

Source: National Heart, Lung, and Blood Institute

fit, and have been fitness walking (moderate to brisk pace) or engaging in a similar exercise (jogging, hiking) for at least 6 months, you can set your goals higher. Go ahead and walk harder and faster, over hill and dale, and rack up your walking mileage—if you're able and willing. But if you've been sedentary or not exercised regularly for some time, you are wise to take it slow.

If one of your goals is to lose weight, remember that the only way to shed pounds is to create a calorie deficit—to burn more calories than you consume. And cutting calories alone won't cut it. To lose it, you've got to move it—and there isn't any way around that. Sharply reducing calories can be harmful to your health and can actually slow down your metabolism. For best and lasting weight loss, eat a balanced diet and exercise regularly.

FitnessFACT
Best Tact: Slow Burn

Experts agree that for most people losing 1 to 2 pounds a week is the most sensible and effective rate of weight loss. Dropping too much too quickly can trick your body into thinking it is being starved and needs to stockpile energy (in the form of fat), which triggers your body to slow your metabolism in an effort to conserve calories.

Also, you actually burn more calories per mile at a slower pace, because you're essentially stopping and starting with each step, whereas with brisk walking, the momentum of your arms swinging and your leg muscles pumping helps you along. However, walking faster uses more muscles and burns more calories per step.

Lifestyle Activity Level Chart

Activity Level	Types of Activities	Steps per day	Calories per hour (daily average)
Sedentary	reading, writing, watching TV or movies, playing video games, knitting, scrap-booking, office work, driving	Under 3,000	80-100
Light	strolling short distance, cooking, doing dishes, showering, dusting, folding clothes, taking out trash	3,000-6,000	110-160
Moderate	walking, making bed, vacuuming, washing car, golf, shopping, gardening, light carpentry, childcare	6,000-10,000	170-240
Active	brisk walking, hiking, climbing stairs, yoga, Pilates, shoveling, scrubbing, biking, package delivery, construction	10,000-12,500	250-400
Very Active	speed walking, jogging, high-impact aerobics, weightlifting, 250-400mountain biking, rowing, competitive sports	12,500-15,000	400+

FitnessFACT

Age: Not Just an Attitude

If you're thin and one of your goals is to build muscle, you'll need to exercise more often and more strenuously, and you'll need to create a caloric excess (consume more than you burn) or at least sustain a caloric balance (burn no more than you consume).

If you want to either slim down or beef up, keep in mind that these changes may take a while to see in the mirror. Be assured that as you follow this program and consistently work toward 10,000 steps a day, positive changes will take place inside your body. Your body composition will improve. Your energy, strength, and flexibility will increase. Meanwhile, your health risks will decrease. You will lose weight and gain muscle. Just keep moving forward, a few steps at a time, a day at a time.

Exercise is shown to decrease the effects of and slow the rate of aging. Even if you're young at heart and do all the right things to stay fit, though, your physical capacity (exertion and stamina) diminishes as you age. Generally, at age 50 your physical capacity will be about 70% of what it was at 25, and at 70 it will be about 50%. Something to take into account when setting your exercise goals.

Even when the physical results aren't immediately obvious, simply recording each day's steps in your Daily Log will give you concrete evidence that you are making progress, that you are increasing your daily activity, that you are doing something positive to manage your weight and to live a healthier, happier, and longer life.

Fidget While You Work

Did you know you can increase your physical activity level without taking a single step? The Mayo Clinic has identified a link between being lean and how much you fidget, stand, sit, and recline throughout your typical day. In measuring the movements of 10 lean and 10 mildly obese volunteers, every half second for 24 hours a day, researchers found that the obese subjects sat for an average of two hours more a day than the lean subjects. They also found that the lean subjects racked up a lot of small movements from fidgeting, pacing, and standing, which burned up to an additional 350 calories a day. For three super-easy ways to bump up your activity level and burn extra calories: (1) stand when you can, (2) sit rather than recline, (3) fidget like there's no one watching.

Complete the Goals Questionnaire, below. Think carefully about your responses to this and to the earlier quizzes in this chapter, and how it all relates to your exercise goals. Then, record your goals in your Daily Step Log. You can use the sample My Step Goals Worksheet, below, as a guide, but make sure to use your own baseline and to set goals that work for you.

Burn, Baby, Burn!

Walking is a sure-fire calorie-burner and fat-buster. Of course, seeing is believing. So take a look at these great results:

- When walking, half of the body's fuel comes from body fat, as compared with less than a third when running.
- Taking 10,000 steps is the rough equivalent of walking 5 miles. A five-mile brisk walk burns about 500 calories.

Walking Level Chart

Walking Level	Fitness Level	Intensity	Pace	Speed	Calories
Beginner	sedentary, extremely overweight or obese	Slow: light exertion, minimal for condition	at own pace		1-2 per minute
Moderate	light activities, exercise 1-3 times a week	Normal: moderate exertion, comfortable breathing & talking	70 per minute	30 minutes per mile (2 mph)	3-4 per minute
Intermediate	active, exercise regularly	Brisk: concentrated exertion, slight difficulty breathing & talking	105 per minute	20 minutes per mile (3 mph)	5-6 per minute
Advanced	very active for at least 6 months, excellent physical condition	Fast: heavy exertion, labored breathing, sweating, difficulty talking	140 per minute	15 minutes per mile (4 mph)	7-10 per minute

- Walking briskly for one mile—about 2,000 steps—consumes 100 calories. Burning an extra 100 calories a day will help the average person lose about 10 pounds a year.
- A moderately heavy person who takes a brisk 10-minute walk every day burns about 250 calories a week, resulting in a potential weight loss of about 4 pounds a year.
- A 150 pound person burns about 100 calories per mile. Picking up the pace can double the calories used per minute.

Go for the Goals Questionnaire

Earlier in this chapter, you identified your why for exercising. Now it's time to zero in on your primary objectives, which are directly linked to your exercise goals. So, once again, grab a pen or pencil and some blank paper (or write in the book) and answer these simple questions. If more than one multiple-choice answer applies, either check all that apply or number your responses in order of their importance to you. Skip any question that does not apply.

With this exercise program, I hope to:

___ Look better   ___ Feel better

___ Be healthier   ___ Get leaner / reduce excess fat on my body to _____%.

___ Lose weight. How much? _____ lbs.

___ Lose inches. Where and how many:

         chest _____   arms _____   waist _____

         hips _____   thighs _____   calves _____

___ Manage my weight (stop gaining / prevent from gaining)

___ Build muscle   ___ Improve my muscle tone and body shape

___ Increase my body strength   ___ Increase my physical stamina

___ Increase my coordination and flexibility (decrease stiffness)

___ Increase my energy

___ Reduce stress / improve my mood / boost my spirits

___ Have fun / enjoy myself   ___ Compete in an athletic event

___ Reduce the aches and pains in my joints, muscles, bones

___ Reduce or manage my cholesterol   ___ Reduce or manage my blood pressure

___ Reduce my risk of chronic illness. Specify those you are most concerned about:

         ___ diabetes   ___ cardiovascular disease

         ___ high blood pressure   ___ stroke

         ___ osteoporosis   ___ arthritis

         ___ gall bladder disease   ___ colon cancer

         ___ other _____

__ Slow down the aging process
__ Extend my life
__ Provide a good example for my children and/or spouse

Sample Step Goals Worksheet: Level One

Baseline: 6,000 steps per day Level One Goals
90-Day Goal: Add 4,000 exercise steps per day = 10,000 total steps per day

	Duration	Exercise Steps per day	Total Steps per day (baseline + exercise)
Week 1	10 minutes	1,000	7,000
Week 2	10 minutes	1,000	7,000
Week 3	10 minutes	1,000	7,000
Week 4	20 minutes	2,000	8,000
Week 5	20 minutes	2,000	8,000
Week 6	20 minutes	2,000	8,000
Week 7	30 minutes	3,000	9,000
Week 8	30 minutes	3,000	9,000
Week 9	30 minutes	3,000	9,000
Week 10	40 minutes	4,000	10,000
Week 11	40 minutes	4,000	10,000
Week 12	40 minutes	4,000	10,000

Note: These figures are based on a moderate to brisk walking pace averaging about 100 steps a minute. For simplicity, the figures are rounded off; we suggest you do the same when setting your goals.

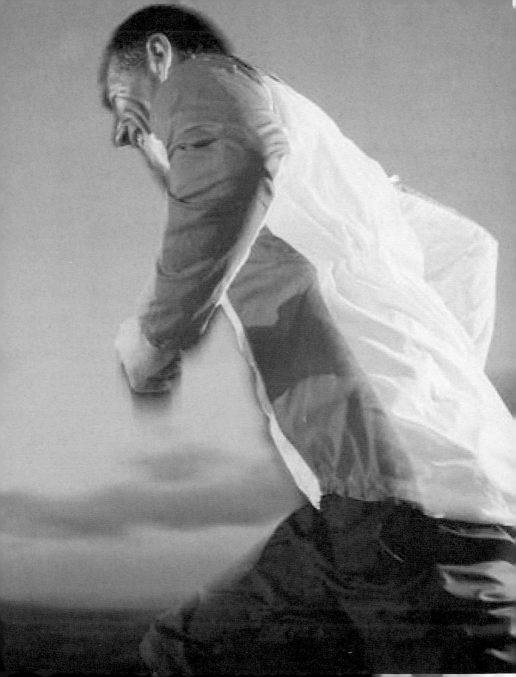

lose one in the dryer, you'll always have a match for it.

Do-Right Duds

Another bonus of walking is that you don't have to buy special clothing or hassle with changing out of your regular clothes to do it. And you'll never have to worry about feeling like a frump, working out next to the Adonis in his muscle-shirt or the living Barbie doll squeezed into the latest (and most revealing) Lycra fitness get-up. As long as your clothing is comfortable, breathes, and fits properly (droopy drawers might be hip in certain circles, but tripping over your pants cuff isn't), anything goes. Jeans, khakis, sweatpants, shorts, skorts, even skirts (or kilts, for ye Celtic dudes out there)—whatever suits your fashion fancy.

Clothing should be loose-fitting enough that it doesn't cling to your skin, rub flesh, or restrict breathing or circulation, but not so loose that it bunches up, allows inclement weather to reach the body, or drags on the ground. The best fabric for walking apparel is one that will draw (wick) sweat away from your body, which will keep you dry and your body temperature more even. As comfortable as cotton might be, it retains sweat and impedes evaporation, making you hot and clammy in warm weather and cold and clammy in cool weather. So, it is best to stay away from cotton or go with a cotton-synthetic blend. To

>>**tip**

Give your new walking shoes a 2- to 3-day trial run indoors on a clean, preferably soft surface. That way, you won't scuff them up outside and can exchange them, in the event they don't work for you.

keep laundry expenses to a minimum and for your convenience, it is also wise to select washable clothing.

For indoor walking (for example, treadmill or circling a mall), you will be most comfortable in lightweight, breathable, wicking material, such as silk, Coolmax, microfiber, polyester, or a cotton-polyester blend.

For outdoor walking, always dress for the weather. Make sure not to overdress in warm weather or to be caught ill-suited for inclement weather.

For sunny days, make sure to protect yourself with sunglasses; a visor, baseball cap, or sun hat; and sun block.

If the weather is cool, wet, or variable, dress in thin layers: a base layer of lightweight, breathable fabric; an insulating layer of fleece, pile, wool, or down (for ultra-cold days); and an outer layer made of a water-resistant and/or windproof material that breathes, such as Goretex or Ultrex, or simply a rain slicker or windbreaker, if it will keep you dry and warm enough. That way, as you walk and your body temperature rises or the weather improves, you can peel off the outer and insulating layer, as needed, to suit your comfort level. Using lightweight garments makes it easier for you to tie them around your waist or shoulders.

Anatomy of a Good Walking Shoe

Not all walking shoes are created equal. A shoe that will give you sufficient comfort, support, protection, and durability will have the following features.

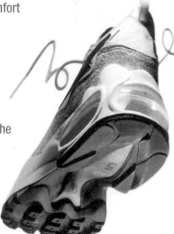

- A rounded toe box to prevent blisters and calluses
- A low, rounded (or beveled), reinforced heel for comfort and support
- An Achilles notch to reduce stress on the Achilles tendon
- Thick insole that conforms to the shape of your foot to support and cushion the arch
- Strong but lightweight and breathable material on the "upper" to hold the shoe snugly on the foot, to protect skin against injury, and to keep feet cool and ventilated
- A gel pad between the insole and the outer sole to minimize impact when the foot hits the ground
- A roller ball beneath the gel pad and positioned properly under the arch to stabilize your stride if your foot tends to roll inward when striking the ground (as many people's feet do when walking)
- An outer sole with moderate tread for good traction without the more intense physical exertion that a heavier tread (as in trail or running shoes) requires
- Laces that stay tied and are not too short or too long, to prevent tripping on untied shoelaces and injuries caused when shoes are too loose

Finding Your Arch-Type

Not many people know that humans actually have two types of arches: longitudinal (lengthwise) and metatarsal (side-to-side). The arches in your feet are a complex configuration of bones, muscles, ligaments, and tendons that have a tremendous impact on how you walk. As you walk, both of these spring-loaded, flexible arches help distribute your body weight even across each of your feet.

There are three basic types of arches, and selecting a shoe that is appropriate for your arch type will ensure your comfort, reduce the risk of injury, and enhance your stride when walking.

In cold weather, you might want to slip on a pair of gloves and a knit cap that covers your head, ears, and neck. Sunglasses and sun block might also be warranted on cool, dry days.

The Beat Goes On

Music may soothe the savage beast, but it can also motivate the indolent couch slug. Walkmans or MP3 players (such as the iPod) can stave off one of the greatest enemies of any exercise: boredom. Studies have shown that music can help you keep trucking. Scientists at the Sport Science Department at Lincoln College in the United Kingdom found that subjects walked significantly longer when listening to either familiar or unfamiliar music than when listening to white noise. The subjects rated the familiar music as being more motivating, but the improvements in endurance were the same when listening to both the new and familiar tunes.

To find your arch type:

Dip your foot in water, step on a piece of cardboard, and then step off the cardboard. If you can see most of your foot on the paper, you probably have low arches. If you see very little of your foot, you probably have high arches.

Low Arch (flat feet)	Tendency to roll inward, which can stress muscles and joints in your feet and knees. Look for a walking shoe with motion control (such as a roller ball) to help stabilize your foot.
High Arch	Reduces the foot's shock absorbency, which puts excessive strain on joints and muscles. Look for a walking shoe with sufficient arch cushioning to compensate for your inadequate arch
Neutral Arch	Not overly flat or overly arched. Look for shoes with a firm midsole, straight or semicurved "lasts" (shape of the footprint the shoe is built around), and moderate rear-foot stability

Motivation is not the only performance-boosting aspect that music provides. It is also a source of distraction, in a good way. At the Department of Movement and Sport Sciences at Ghent University in Belgium, researchers examined 30 severely obese youngsters who ran on a treadmill until exhaustion. The subjects ran significantly longer when music was played than when they

>>tip

These Suits Aren't Made for Walkin'

No doubt you've heard the phrase "dress for success." When it comes to increasing your daily activity and burning calories, it is a fact. A study by the American Council on Exercise found that people who wore more casual clothes to work were more active during the day. All of the subjects were outfitted with step counters, and the people who wore jeans took 8% more steps than those in work attire (must be the starch in the suits). If you have the opportunity, wear lighter, looser, more casual clothing to work, and you could chalk up an extra quarter-mile a day.

performed the same test in silence. Scientists theorized that when the kids were distracted by music, it took longer for them to perceive bodily discomforts and decide to stop running.

When choosing your music, try to find songs that have a number-of-beats-per-minute that is similar to the rhythm of your walking stride. Also, songs with an upbeat tempo and positive lyrics will provide a more effective accompaniment to your walking than slow, soothing, and sad tunes.

Safety should always be a priority when listening to music while walking. Never wear headphones and always keep the volume low enough for you to hear approaching vehicles, people, and animals as well as any other audible "danger" signals (such as brakes screeching or limbs cracking). In high-traffic areas or unfamiliar neighborhoods, always turn the music off in favor of being tuned in to your surroundings.

Prodigal Sun

Regular sun exposure is vital for your health, sleep, and mood. But it can be too much of a good thing. The negative effects of excessive sun exposure, from freckles to skin cancer, don't come only from immediate contact with searing rays. It can also come from slow and gradual exposure, day by day, even when the sky is overcast. Plus, UV rays can penetrate right through clothing, to varying degrees.

Some specialty brands of clothing now have a Sun Protection Factor (SPF) rating on their shirts, pants, shorts, and hats. As a rule, dark colors offer more protection than lighter ones, and tightly woven fibers provide more protection than loosely woven clothing. If you can see light through a fabric, UV rays can penetrate it.

Your scalp is ripe for skin cancers, so wearing a hat is a smart choice. A brimmed hat works best, because skin cancers commonly develop on the back of the neck or the ears, places where a baseball cap offers no protection.

With what we now know about the dangers of overexposure to the sun's harmful rays and with the depletion of the UV-filtering ozone layer, this should go without saying: Always wear sunscreen. It should have an SPF rating of at least 15— higher if you are fair-skinned, have had skin cancer or pre-cancer cells, spend a lot of time outdoors, or take certain medications or supplements (check with your doctor). The SPF represents the degree to which the sunscreen decreases your resistance to the sun's harmful rays. For example, when wearing a sunscreen with SPF 30, a half hour (30 minutes) in the sun is equivalent to one unprotected minute—a resistance of 30:1. Make sure to apply sunscreen 20 to 30 minutes before going outside, so your skin has time to absorb it, and to reapply it as recommended on the manufacturer's label or by your doctor.

>>tip

Time ▌Your Time in the Sun

Just like you can check the weather and air quality for your area on a daily basis, you can now check the UV Index in your local newspaper or on the Internet (www.cpc.ncep.noaa.gov). On days with a high UV Index, especially if you are at risk for skin cancers, you may want to plan walks or hikes for early in the morning or later in the evening, staying out of the sun between 10:00 A.M. and 4:00 P.M., when harmful rays are at their highest concentration.

Night Walker

Many people enjoy taking their strolls at night. There is less smog, fewer particles in the air, and the temperature can be more pleasant than when the sun is blazing. If you are a nocturnal strider, walk in a well-lit and familiar place, preferably with a partner or group, and invest in some reflective garments or put some reflective stickers or safety bands on your clothing.

The University of Michigan Transportation Research Institute recently conducted an experiment that gauged drivers' reactions to nighttime pedestrians. The results showed that when pedestrians crossed the road without wearing reflective gear, drivers noticed them at a distance of 35 meters. When the walkers wore reflective items on their torso, the drivers saw them 136 meters away. The distance jumped to 241 meters when pedestrians wore reflective items on their ankles or wrists.

Don't worry; you don't have to look like a science experiment just to be safe. Reflective materials are often designed discretely and attractively into athletic shoes and clothing. You can also buy reflective strips that use Velcro to attach onto your own walking clothes.

H20 Yeah!

It never hurts to drink a glass of water before you start walking, but walking on a dry tank can harm you. Keeping hydrated is vital to your body's ability to control its temperature and a balanced electrolyte level. Dehydration can cause fatigue, dizziness, muscle cramps, nausea, overheating, and heat stroke.

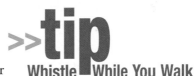

>>tip
Whistle While You Walk
Or sing. Both whistling and singing will enhance your breathing, muscle tone, and relaxation as you stride on down the street. Who cares what the neighbors think?

If drinking an 8- to 10-ounce glass of water leaves you with a sloshing or bloated feeling in your stomach, have half a glass of water 20-30 minutes before your walk and then another half a glass when you return from your walk. If drinking a full glass of water makes you feel queasy, that's an indication you're running on empty and need to eat a healthy snack.

If you're going for a short walk—say, a 10-minute jaunt or once around the block—drink some water before you go and again when you return. For walks of 30 minutes or more, bring along

>>tip

Get Yourself a Partner

Birds of a feather really do stick together—and to their shared walking routines. To increase your enjoyment and safety, find a walking buddy or form a walking group.

some water. As a rule of thumb, your body needs 8 ounces of water for every 15 minutes of exercise.

You'll find a variety of water carriers out there, including those with shoulder straps and those that attach to your waist. Some have containers that you fill with water; others are designed for carrying individual-sized bottled water.

Fuel to Go

Smart snacking is actually good for your health and managing your weight. To efficiently maintain body and brain functions, your body generally needs refueling every 4 hours (during waking hours). So, adding two or three healthy snacks in between your three squares a day is nutritionally wise.

If your walking time happens to coincide with your snacking time, bring along a small portion of an energy-building, rather than a fat-building, food. If you're walking briskly or hiking for more than 60 minutes, you'll need to refuel during your excursion to maintain a healthy blood sugar level.

The best food to bring along in your fanny pack:

• Nuts (almonds, walnuts, and peanuts are best, but any are fine;

> **" Fitness—if it came in a bottle, everybody would have a great body. "**
>
> *—Cher*

unsalted are best)

- Sunflower seeds (shelled and unsalted are best)
- Dried Fruit (apricots, pineapple, cranberries, blueberries, and the old standard, raisins)
- Fresh Fruit and Veggies (whatever turns you on, rinsed thoroughly, organic is best)
- Cheese Sticks (low-fat, such as mozzarella, are best)
- Trail Mix (any combo of seeds, nuts, dried fruits, whole grains; a few M&Ms thrown in won't hurt and will give you a little carb boost)
- Turkey Jerky (or beef, if you prefer)
- Energy Bars (a mix of carbs, protein, and fat; yogurt covered is fine but avoid chocolate-covered)
- Energy Gels (must consume with water)

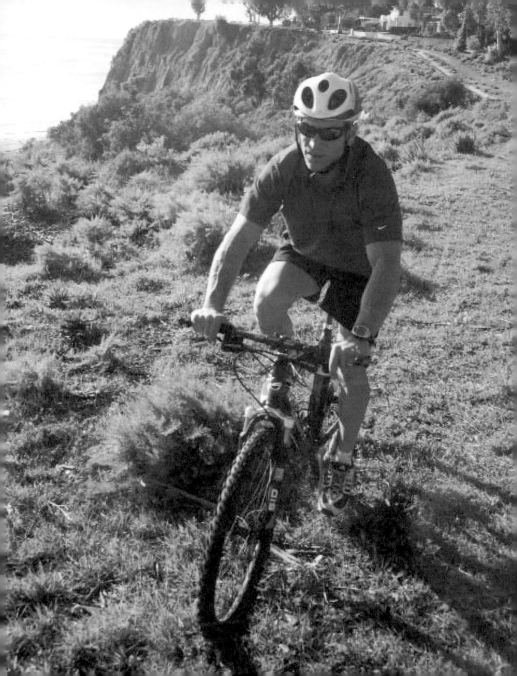

CHAPTER FIVE

GET MOVING
90 Days to a Trimmer, Healthier You

The U.S Surgeon General's call to arms, or rather to the health of the good people of this country, is to shave off 100 calories and add on 30 minutes of exercise (one mile, equivalent to 2,000 steps) each day. That's enough to reduce the risk of chronic diseases. It's probably not enough to lose weight and shape up. So, the goal of the 10,000-Steps-A-Day Program is to help you add at least 30 minutes of fitness walking (specifically for exercise) to your day plus increase the number of steps you take in the normal course of your life—with the end goal of increasing your daily activity to the equivalent of 10,000 steps or more.

As with any goal, the success of your "step your way to fitness" goal relies upon having a plan as well as both the desire and discipline to see it through. Dreamers may have high hopes and plenty of great ideas, but if they lack an action plan and accountability, they're unlikely to get off the ground, much less reach their destination, because they don't have the right guidance system in place to guide and propel them there. Go-getters, on the other hand, may have the zip and good intentions, but if they don't take the time to learn the rules of the game and to develop their own game plan, they're missing the essential what, where, when, why, and how to keep them from going out of bounds, getting injured, and petering out before they reach the goal line.

The 10,000-Steps-A-Day Program gives legs to your fitness dreams—by giving you the basic tools (like your Step-Counter) and support (like your Daily Step Log) to move you consistently toward your goals—one logical, attainable, planned step at a time.

How Much, How Hard, How Fast

The 10,000-Steps-A-Day Program is a six-month program divided into two 90-day courses (12 weeks, 3 months each). The objectives of the first course (Level One) are to: (a) add a regular fitness activity to your life and (b) get you as close to 10,000 steps a day as you are willing and able. The objectives of Level Two (covered in Chapter Seven) are to: (a) help you make fitness walking a habitual part of each day and (b) encourage you to work toward your optimal weight and physical condition.

Both levels involve adding steps to your daily activities and gradually increasing the duration and intensity of your fitness walking (or equivalent exercise activity). Each 12-week course is broken into intervals, starting with a start-up interval of 1 to 2 weeks and then 2-week, 3-week, or 4-week intervals, which you determine based on your personal needs, goals, etc.

We've designed the 10,000-Steps-A-Day Program this way because studies show that:

- The most effective fitness activities are those that become a routine part of your life.
- It usually takes 6 months of doing an exercise before it becomes routine.
- People are more likely to exercise sufficiently and regularly when they have measurable goals and a step-by-step plan for achieving them.

When you think about it, isn't that how much of success in life is achieved? By setting goals, both large and small, and systematically working toward them, taking stock of progress along the way, and making necessary adjustments and accommodations to keep up the forward momentum? Of course it is.

Few things in life are more satisfying than setting out to accomplish something that is meaningful to you and then achieving it— whether that goal is getting a degree, building a career, remodeling a house, launching a business, or raising happy, healthy children. By the same token, the only thing more disappointing than failing to achieve an important personal goal is failing to even try. And in the grand scheme of things, what could be more important than your health?

>>tip

Jabberwalky

You can measure your exertion level while walking with this simple talk test: If you can breathe normally while talking and walking at the same time, you're taking it slow and easy. If your breathing is slightly labored, you're probably clipping along at a moderate pace that is appropriate for most moderately active people without health concerns. If you're too out of breath to carry on a running conversation, you're working intensely—and if you're not a regular exerciser in good fitness condition, you'd better simmer down and slow down.

That is why your health must be your first consideration when selecting appropriate activities and setting a sensible pace for your walking routine. So, armed with all the factors that went into defining your fitness profile in Chapter Three, take a few minutes now to identify walking activities that fit your current physical condition and level of activity (for the last 6-12 months), your lifestyle (how you spend your time), and your interests.

Remember to take into consideration the difficulty and duration of the activity. Walking on rough surfaces (sand, gravel, thick grass), through woodlands or fields, over hills, and up and down stairs is equivalent to a brisk-to-intense walk. If you are obese, sedentary, or have any health concerns, you should avoid long and hard walks. If you haven't exercised regularly for 6 or more months, are overweight, or tire easily, it is best to start out slow and easy. You can always increase the intensity and duration of your walking later, in sensible increments.

Make sure to always wear your Step-Counter, so that you have an accurate measurement of how much you've walked. It can be as easy to underestimate the duration of an activity as it is to overestimate it.

One effective way to plan your daily walking routine is to choose at least three walking activities for each day. That way, if your day doesn't go as planned (as days are wont to do) and you miss any of your planned walking activities, you've still got at least one, if not two, other activities for that day, and you can always increase the duration or intensity to compensate for the missed activity. Next, figure out where you can best fit those activities into your schedule. Then, write it down on your calendar, day planner, or in the Activity Planner section of your Daily Step Log.

A simpler way to plan your walking schedule is to set a goal of a specific number of minutes of walking per day for each of the first 90 days of your 10,000-Steps-A-Day Program. After you've completed Level One, you can then schedule out your minutes-per-day of walking for each of the 90 days of Level Two. Ideally, you should start out with a lower increment, of say 10 or 15 minutes, and gradually build up to a larger number, of say 30-45 minutes. If you're already somewhat physically active, not overweight or obese, and in good health, you can even start out at and work toward higher numbers—say, go from 20 to 60 minutes or 30 to 70 minutes. Again, writing your walking plan in your Daily Step Log (or your regular day planner or calendar) will help motivate you to walk, increasing your odds of reaching your goals.

Sample Activity Planner

Level One

Week 1		Activity	Time	Duration
Mon.	1	Walk dog	7:00 A.M.	15 min.
	2	Walk to sub shop for lunch	Noon	20 min. (round trip)
	3	Walk around mall before buying Mother's Day cards	5:30 P.M.	10 min.
Sun.	1	Walk with hubby to Chubby's for breakfast	9:00 A.M.	30 min. (round)
	2	Push niece in stroller at park	2:00 P.M.	30 min.
	3	Treadmill	6:00 P.M.	10 min.

When to Walk

This is kind of a no-brainer. The best time to walk is whatever time is best for you. Are you an early riser or a night owl? Do you have more energy in the morning, afternoon, or evening? What part of the day is it easiest for you to block out 10 to 30 minutes for walking: before your busy day begins, during your toddler's mid-morning nap, mid-day, late afternoon, immediately after

Mark Your Step

Here are some standard measurements (in steps) of common distance markers, which may vary slightly in your town or neighborhood.

Marker	Steps
City block	155-200
Between streetlights	75
Between fire hydrants	150
Basketball court	48
Football field	150
Baseball diamond	180
Quarter-Mile Track (1 lap)	625
One mile	2,000-2,625

work, early evening, after the kids are down for the night, or, if you work an odd shift, in the middle of the night? At those periods in the day when you are most likely to have the most time and energy for walking, do you have easy access to a comfortable and safe place to walk?

The majority of people claim to prefer exercising in the morning, when they say they feel the most energetic, rested, focused, and "fresh," and before the responsibilities and worries of the day take over their day. Early-morning exercise might not be the way to go for midlifers and seniors, who tend to wake up stiff and sore and need some time to flex and warm muscles and joints and to get their motors running.

Some folks enthusiastically endorse doing their fitness activities in the late afternoon or early evening, after their busy day, when their muscles are warmer, stronger, and more flexible. Many late-day exercisers also claim that they feel the most alert, clear, and energetic then.

FitnessFACT
Walking Takes a Bow Wow

We all know that walking the dog is good for man's best friend. Now there is compelling evidence it is good for the canine's master too.

In a dog-walking study conducted by the College of Veterinary Medicine's Research Center for Human-Animal Interaction at the University of Missouri-Columbia, a group of sedentary, economically disadvantaged people with multiple chronic illnesses were teamed up with loaner companion dogs provided by the Pet Assisted Love and Support (PALS) program. The dog-walkers were divided into two smaller groups: one for a 26-week trial, the other for a 50-week trial. Both groups started by walking 10 minutes a day 3 times a week and gradually worked up to 20 minutes a day 5 days a week. All lost weight, but the 50-week walkers lost more, averaging a weight loss of 14 pounds each. One nearly housebound participant who used an electric scooter to get around her apartment was able to walk to the neighborhood grocery store and back by the end of the 50-week program.

Still other people swear by midday exercise, which provides a welcome respite in the middle of a packed day. Lunch breaks are sometimes the only time working parents can squeeze out of their hectic day, and during winter months, it is their only opportunity to walk outside in daylight. Also, some prefer midday exercising because, by nature, they are slow risers in the morning, experience an energy dip in the late afternoon, or hit the wall in the evening.

If you're looking for experts to give you a pat answer on when is the most effective time to exercise, you may be surprised to learn that most of their answers will be pretty much the same: It depends … on you and your day, because every body is unique and every day your body functions a little differently. It all depends on your "circadian rhythms"—the patterns of your body's various functions during any given 24-hour cycle. An internal pacemaker within the brain sends signals throughout the body to keep more than 100 different rhythms—such as body temperature, heart rate, blood pressure, lung capacity, energy levels, and pain threshold—on their individual time cycles. So, depending on your natural circadian rhythms and on the external things that can alter them, such as sleep, activity, diet, medications, and stress—there will likely be certain times of the day when exercise feels better to you and works better for you. There will be times when life's challenges throw your rhythm off a few beats, and you might need to temporarily or even permanently (for example, as you age) change your exercise routine accordingly.

You don't need to understand the complex physiology of circadian rhythms and their effect on exercise to safely proceed and succeed in your 10,000-Steps-A-Day-Program. All you really need to know is that eating, sleeping, and exercising properly will help to prevent disruptions in your circadian rhythms. In fact, maintaining a regular exercise routine can actually help to keep your body in sync.

>>tip

Grab Your Partner, Go-Go-Go!

Having a walking partner or being part of a walking group yields several benefits. It increases your enjoyment, gives you something to look forward to, and helps to ward off boredom. Just the accountability factor alone—not wanting to disappoint your walking buddies—will help to keep you hoofing it. Plus, good walking partner(s) encourage and support one another. Consequently, you are motivated to walk more often and more regularly. Plus, there is always more safety in numbers. Just make sure to select a partner or group with a fitness level, walking goals, schedule, and interests similar to yours.

Speaking of exercise schedules, now is a good time to focus on yours.

Carpe Diem! Seize the Walking-Friendly Minutes of Your Day

Answering these simple questions will help you to schedule walking right into your life:

1. What are your goals for the first leg (90 days) of your personalized 10,000-A-Day Program?

2. How many additional steps (or minutes of walking) per day do you plan to add during your first interval (1 or 2 weeks) and for each of the succeeding intervals (2-week, 3-week, or 4-week) of your 12-week plan?

3. Do you plan to add all of the additional daily steps (or minutes) in a single session—for example, one 30-minute (2,000 steps) walk—or in two or more smaller sessions, of, say, 10-minutes or 15-minutes each?

FitnessFACT

Swamped

The most time-crunched Americans are 30 to 45 years old, work 40-plus hours a week, and are the parents of young children, according to numerous time studies.

4. At what times of the day do you feel the most rested, energetic, and relaxed?

5. At what times of the day do you feel the most tired, stressed, and crunched for time?

6. How many hours (or minutes) of "free" time do you have each day? Be specific, identifying any variances from day to day and between weekdays and weekends.

7. How do you currently use your free time? Again, be specific, accounting for when and how long you spend in each activity.

8. Which leisure activities are you willing and able to do less of or replace with walking (or an equivalent physical activity)? Remember, this is not about giving up all of your down time and play time; everyone needs a daily dose of R&R. Just look for 10-, 15-, 20-, and 30-minute pockets in your day when you can swap a leisure activity (or a few) with walking.

9. Based on your lifestyle, your schedule, and your body's natural circadian rhythms, when are the most ideal and realistic time(s) of the day for you to walk? Name at least three different blocks of time.

FitnessFACT

The Air Out There

If you suffer from asthma, allergies, or chemical sensitivities, always carry your inhaler with you when walking outside or indoors where dust, mold, and chemicals might be present (stores, airports, office buildings). It is also best not to walk when the air-quality is poor (high levels of smog, smoke, pollen, or particulates), especially at dusk, when cool air pushes these air-borne contaminants to street level.

Where to Walk

In a word: anywhere! As long as the site is safe for walking and for your health, you can take your 10-minute, 15-minute, 20-minute, 30-minute or more walk—whatever interval you've set as your starting goal—indoors or outside. At a park or inside a mall. Around the block or around a sports track. At a community center, the Y, or your gym. Near your home or your place of employment—for that matter, in your home or office building—or any convenient point in between.

The nearer your walking place is to where you normally are and the routes you typically travel in your everyday life, the more likely you are to actually walk there on a consistent basis … usually. Some of us prefer and might even need a change of place to change our pace. Sometimes, taking yourself out of your element—away from your home, your job, your neighborhood—and walking in an environment that is beautiful, peaceful, or stimulating gives you the incentive to walk more and more often. Others use special out-of-the-way walking excursions—whether nature hikes, big-city walking tours, window shopping jaunts, or a round of golf—on weekends, holidays, or as a monthly reward for managing to squeeze daily walking into their hectic schedules.

All it takes is a little forethought and planning, and some slight changes to your daily habits. Creativity also goes a long way, too, in mapping out walking routines that will keep your interest level high and tediousness at bay. But let's not forget the power of spontaneity to move that body. You never know when an opportunity to slip in an extra few minutes or a few hundred more steps worth of walking might present itself, and if your eyes and mind are open to such possibilities, you'll be poised to take advantage of them.

Walking Strategies to Live By

There must be 50 ways to easily add a walk or two to your day. Make that 100 ways. Probably more. Here are just a few.

- Replace your coffee or smoking break with a 10-minute walking break.

When Not to Move It to Lose It

As a rule of thumb, avoid brisk, vigorous, or long-duration walks when:

- The environment (whether indoors or outdoors) is too hot
- The environment is too cold
- You've eaten a heavy meal
- Your blood sugar is low
- You are fatigued or sleep-deprived
- You are dehydrated
- You have an injury that limits your physical activity (check with your doctor)
- You are under the weather (including colds and stomach flu)

On the other hand, slow to moderate-intensity walks of short duration (less than 30 minutes) are perfectly safe under these conditions and can even be helpful, with the exception of people who are obese or have a chronic illness.

- Meet a friend at a park for a 30-minute chat-and-stride, rather than for happy hour. Or, if you're determined to have that wine and cheese or nachos and beer, go to happy hour afterward, and if you're pressed for time, walk for 10 or 15 minutes instead of 30.
- If you park in a public garage separate from your office, choose one a few blocks away.
- When your child tries your patience, rather than giving her or him a time-out, give yourself one by taking both of you for a short walk. Not only will you get in some extra steps, but you'll be amazed at how a little exercise and fresh air can turn an unruly or upset little one into a little angel.
- Walk the dog. Walk longer with your dog; take an extra lap around the dog park. If you don't have a dog, borrow one. People are always looking for fill-in dog walkers; surely you have friends and neighbors with pets who would be more than willing to lend you're their pooch.
- Before shopping, take a steady saunter around the inside perimeter of the entire mall, without stopping at any of the stores and staying to the far right to get in the maximum distance. As a side benefit, you can window-shop as you go to spot any great buys and must-haves you might otherwise have missed.

FitnessFACT

"Habitual exercisers" begin each day expecting and planning to engage in physical activity, according to Russ Pate, a professor of exercise science at the University of South Carolina who was a member of the committee that developed the Revised Dietary Guidelines for Americans, issued by the U.S. Department of Health and Human Services, which recommends at least 30 minutes of daily exercise. They sort of mentally "scan through their day" first thing in the morning to figure out the best time to exercise. And they make exercise a priority, not allowing non-emergencies to interfere with their exercise. Even when physical activities get bumped by necessity, they simply rearrange their schedule to fit it in somewhere else.

- If you use a taxi or public transportation, get out a block or one stop early and hoof it the rest of the way to your destination. Or walk a block or two before hailing a cab.
- Brownbag it (with healthy foods, of course) and spend 10 or 15 minutes of your lunch break at work walking rather than the entire 30 or 60 minutes munching and slouching.
- When going out to lunch at work, choose a restaurant within walking distance and chalk up additional steps in both directions.
- While watching your kid's (or any) sports event, circle the field (or court, or track, or course) as you watch and cheer them on, rather than just sitting on the sidelines.
- While waiting for an incoming or outgoing plane, walk around the airport rather than sitting and reading the newspaper,

watching a video or playing a video game on your laptop, people watching, or snoozing. With all the flight delays and protracted check-in procedures, you've got to be there so far ahead of time these days, you might as well put the time to good-for-you use.

- At the beach or at the lake, don't just lie there soaking in the rays or sit there watching the boats and the Frisbees sail by. Take a walk in the sand or on the boardwalk.

- Substitute that second helping, dessert, or after-dinner drink with a refreshing post-meal stroll.

- When you need to speak with a co-worker in private, rather than doing it behind closed doors, suggest a walk-and-talk around the building's exterior, parking lot, or commons (if you're fortunate to work on a campus with such a park-like area).

- Walk your child to school, if it's within walking distance, which gives you double the steps and a little time to yourself (or with your spouse or any younger children) when you walk back.

- While waiting for your clothes to wash or dry, walk around the Laundromat or around your block.

- Get your news on the move. Rather than plopping in front of the TV for your early morning or early evening news fix, walk with your Walkman tuned to a news program on your favorite radio station. An added upside: most radio stations broadcast news on the hour and some on the half hour.

Top Ten Rules of the Road

Here are a few safety tips for walking outside.

1. Walk facing traffic, so you can see approaching vehicles in time to get out of the way if necessary
2. Use sidewalks when possible
3. Cross streets carefully and legally (no jay-walking)
4. Avoid hills and rough surfaces if you've been inactive for 6 months or more
5. Walk with a partner or group after dark, in unfamiliar locations, and in places that might put you at risk of personal crime (assault, robbery)
6. Wear light-colored clothing, preferably with reflective material, at dawn, dusk, and after dark
7. Wear your Step-Counter and a watch to make sure you'll know when to head back, so you won't overdo
8. Wear good walking shoes and socks to ensure against blisters and foot injuries
9. Carry identification, a cell phone and/or whistle, and if you walk for 30 minutes or more, water to keep you hydrated and a healthy snack in case your blood sugar drops too low
10. Leave your valuables at home or locked in the trunk of your car, desk, tool box, or gym locker

• Exchange a 30-minute family TV show for a walk with your children. A nearby playground, park, or school will provide a safe place for your kids to walk. (But don't let them go alone.) If it's within easy walking distance, you can score extra steps by walking there and back. Plus, you can play with your kids, chocking up even more steps on your Step-Counter.

Fuel Up

Always make sure you are adequately hydrated before you begin any exercise activity, including just 10 minutes of walking. If you go for a walk first thing in the morning, when you're body is typically low on hydration or dehydrated, it is smart to drink an 8-ounce glass of water before a 10- to 20-minute walk and 10-16 ounces of water if you plan to walk 30 or more minutes.

Avoid drinking coffee, tea, and other diuretics, which actually accelerate dehydration. Also avoid beverages and foods that are loaded with processed sugar, such as soda, fruit juices, pastries, and candy, which cause sharp upswings and then sudden drops in blood sugar, resulting in dizziness, fatigue, and nausea.

There is some evidence that, if you want to lose weight, exercising with little or no food in your stomach increases the amount of stored fat that your body consumes during the physical activity. It does not increase your metabolism, however. Some health experts recommend not exercising on an empty stomach, claiming it poses health risks, such as sudden drops in blood sugar, dizziness, and fatigue, which also increase the risk of injury. If you have diabetes, low or high blood sugar, hypertension, thyroid problems, or liver disease, you should never exercise on an empty stomach. But for most healthy, moderately active people, it is usually okay to walk for up to 30 minutes on an empty stomach, as long as you experience no negative effects during or after your walk.

Most people who exercise regularly as well as most health and exercise specialists recommend not exercising on either a full or an empty stomach. How much and how soon you eat before engaging in walking or any fitness activity depends, in part, on the duration and intensity of the activity. Here are some general guidelines:

1 hour before exercise	small, easy-to-digest snack (banana, nuts, yogurt) 200-300 calories
1-2 hours before exercise	light, easy-to-digest meal or liquid nutrition (yogurt, cottage cheese, protein shakes, smoothies, cup cereal with fruit) 300-400 calories
2-3 hours before exercise	small, lean meal (balance of protein and carbohydrates) 400-500 calories
3-4 hours before exercise	large or heavy meal 600 or more calories

Of course, a nice long walk after a meal will aid in digestion and burn some extra calories.

Warm Up, Cool Down

To stretch or not to stretch: Is that the question? Apparently, according to some exercise physiologists. Actually, the debate is not so much whether to stretch as it is when to stretch. One side of the debate says, "Stretch before fitness walking." The other side says, "Warm up your muscles, then stretch, then walk." One thing both sides do agree on is that stretching after fitness walking (30 minutes or more of moderate, brisk, or speed walking) is a wise move.

There is convincing evidence that stretching cold muscles can injure them. So, if you decide to stretch first, do a few slow and gentle stretches, with no bouncing or protracted "poses."

The easiest and probably the most effective warm up is simply to take an easy pace for the first 3 to 5 minutes of your walk. Slowing it down for the last 3 to 5 minutes is also beneficial, allowing your body to cool down and settle down. Sudden halts to intense exercise can be a shock to the system, which can be uncomfortable at best, and at worst can result in any number of unpleasant consequences, from muscle cramping to cardiovascular irregularities (particularly if there is any underlying health problems).

Another warm up (and cool down) option is to walk in place for 2 to 3 minutes and then do a few minutes of gentle calisthenics, such as leg lifts and windmills.

Stretching after your daily walking exercise not only settles your body down, it also will yield long-term benefits. Regular stretching will help you enjoy:

• Increased flexibility and range of motion in your joints and muscles
• Better posture
• Physical and mental relaxation
• Decreased tension and soreness in your muscles

Warm-up Calisthenics

To help warm up your body before cardiovascular exercise, do a few minutes of these simple exercises. Make sure to do a few minutes of walking in place first.

Arm Circles. Stand erect (do not lock knees), extend arms out to both sides (like a scarecrow), and slowly make large circles with your arms, doing 10 circles forward and then 10 backward.

Leg Swings. Stand sideways next to a sturdy support you can hold on to (such as a table). Swing one leg forward and then back in one smooth, continuous, slow motion. Do 5 to 10 times for each leg.

Trunk Twists. Stand with a wide stance. Lift your arms out to your sides to shoulder height, with elbows slightly bent. Looking straight ahead and keeping your arms extended out to your side, slowly turn as far left as you can and then as far right as you can, going side-to-side 5 to 15 times.

Cool-Down Stretches

Perform these stretches after your fitness walk (30 or more minutes of brisk to intense walking) or equivalent exercise activity—after your muscles are warm. Move slowly into each stretch, hold for 10 to 30 seconds, and then gently release. Remember not to bounce while you are stretching and be sure to breathe! If it starts to hurt, back off. These stretches should not feel painful.

Arm Cross. Stand with your right arm slightly flexed and positioned horizontally across your body. With your left hand, grasp just above the right elbow and gently pull your arm across your chest. Repeat with your left arm.

Straddle. Sit on the floor in a "butterfly" position with your knees bent and pointed outward and the soles of your feet facing in. Bend from the waist and extend your arms forward. Avoid rounding your shoulders.

Knee Flex. Lying on your back, bring your right leg up by flexing your knee and hip. Gently pull your thigh toward your chest and hold. Now repeat with your left leg.

Wall Stretch. Stand facing a wall with your feet set as wide as your shoulders and your toes about a foot from the wall. Lean forward and put your palms on the wall. Step your right foot back about two feet and flex your left knee. Slowly straighten your right leg and lower your heel to the floor. Repeat with your left foot back.

Walk This Way

A walk by any name is a walk. And it isn't rocket science. Yet, one of the biggest mistakes inexperienced fitness walkers make is pushing too hard too soon or simply striding the wrong way. You will get better results and prevent injuries by heeding the following basic walking do's and don'ts.

The Perfect Step

Walking is as second-nature as breathing. But not all of us walk properly, in keeping with the way in which the human body is designed and to prevent excessive wear and tear on the body. The ideal step goes something like this:

The muscles of the lower torso tense, tightening the stomach, tucking the buttocks slightly under, and tipping the pelvis slightly forward as the hip flexes and lifts the leg and swings it forward. The ankle flexes at a 45-degree angle from the ground; toes are pointed forward. The heel touches down directly in front of the body, and the weight of the body rolls forward onto the ball and pushes off from the toes to begin the next step.

> **"** *I'm convinced from the research that a sedentary lifestyle kills you, and moderate activity like walking can be lifesaving. A little exercise is better than none, but more is better than a little.* **"**

–JoAnn Manson, M.D.

Walking Dos

Stand tall. With spine erect and shoulders squared but relaxed. Watch out for sway back or hump back; bad posture

Head up. Chin parallel to the ground; head straight (not tilted left, right, forward, or back).

Eyes forward. Look 15 to 20 feet ahead of you; if you need to look down closer to where you are stepping, lower your eyes and not your whole head.

Elbows bent. At slightly less than a 90-degree angle and kept close to the torso.

Relaxed hands. Loosely closed.

Arms swing naturally. The right arm should swing forward as your left leg swings forward, and the left arm should swing forward as the right leg swings forward.

Butt tucked, tummy tensed. Contract stomach, hip, and buttocks muscles to tip pelvis slightly forward and to walk from the hip flexors rather than the thighs.

Ankle flexed. With toes pointed upward at about 45 degrees.

Step down heel, ball, toes. Lead with your heel, roll forward onto ball, push off with toes.

Walking Don'ts

Do not overextend your stride.

Do not overexert.

Do not scrunch or slump your shoulders.

Do not clench your fists.

Do not lock your knees.

Do not swing your arms in an exaggerated manner.

Do not look at the ground.

Do not use hand or ankle weights unless you are an advanced exerciser.

Do not walk at a speed or intensity that feels uncomfortable to you.

Simple Ways to Add Steps to Your Daily Activities

Almost every activity you do involves at least a few steps. Some involve a lot of steps. At the end of the day, they all add up. Here are 10 easy ways to rack up more steps on your Step-Counter:

>>tip
Sticks and Poles Will Aid Your Goals

For better balance (especially for walkers with injuries or "of a certain age"), use a walking stock or trekking poles. The lightweight poles, which you can find at most sporting-goods stores, give you the added benefit of an enhanced upper-body workout. So does a walking stick, but to a lesser degree. Similar to cross-country skiing, when you step forward with your left foot, you move your right arm forward (keeping the pole lifted slightly so that the handle is about even with your lower ribs) and plant the pole in the ground parallel to your left heel. This works the muscles in your abs, arms, and chest and reduces the stress on your knees. Make sure to use the right size pole (or to adjust it to the right size): You should be able to grip the pole and keep your forearm level as you walk.

1. Park in a space at the section of the parking lot farthest from the door.

2. Take the stairs rather than use the elevator.

3. Go talk to your co-worker rather than e-mailing or calling.

4. Play tag, hide and seek, or Red Rover with your kids.

5. Skip the drive-thru and go inside the bank, dry cleaners, or restaurant.

6. Visit a museum.

7. Go out dancing.

8. Mow the grass.

9. Go to the farmer's market or a flea market.

10. Go to a boat show or home and garden expo.

It All Counts

Let's not forget the energy we burn doing our household chores. To name but a few:

Activity	Steps per minute
Chopping wood	155
Gardening (moderate)	114
Mowing lawn	135
Shoveling snow	155
Vacuuming	85
Washing car	72

Track Your Progress

An exercise journal is the perfect companion to your Step-Counter, and will bring you benefits long after you've completed the six-month 10,000-Steps-A-Month Program.

You can start with the Daily Step Log at the back of this book and purchase a snazzier exercise journal later. Many successful walkers buy a new 12-month journal every year to keep track of their daily steps (or minutes of walking). Others simply record their exercise

FitnessFACT

Midlife women who walk at least 3 hours a week have a 40% lower risk of heart attack and stroke, according to an eight-year study of 84,000 female nurses aged 40-65. Those who walk briskly have a 54% lower risk. Even those who walked at a slower pace had a 32% lower risk of heart disease compared with those who don't walk at all. The proof is in the pudding: Any number of steps at any pace is better—much better—than no steps at all.

goals, schedule, and progress in the same day planners they use for all the other activities in their lives.

To ensure the success of your 10,000-Steps-A-Day Program, make sure to jot down your total steps for the day (as tracked on your Step-Counter) before you go to bed each night. Feel free to also include any exercise-related details, such as if you did a fitness walk or other exercise activity that day, had an exceptionally busy day, didn't feel well, or didn't eat as wisely as you could have. At the end of the week, add up the steps for all seven days and write down your weekly total.

Daily Step Log

Week 1	Total Steps	Exercise Minutes
Mon.	4,623	40

Notes: Great day! Walked Fido in new dog park and found a new walking partner. Plus got in 10 minutes on the treadmill while watching the news.

Sun.	3,009	10

Notes: Slammed with the flu today, but managed to walk the dog to the corner and back.

Total steps this week: _____

Average steps per day: _____

(total steps ÷ 7)

By committing your numbers to paper, you are creating a trail you can constantly refer to in order to keep yourself on track. If you are planning to build up to a number, it will be necessary to record your progress. If you are more casual about your steps, a quick look at your journal can enlighten you to any ruts or stagnation that you may have fallen into. A good journal is also your own personal cheerleader, as you will feel encouraged when you look back at the early days and see how much progress you have made.

Now, go on! Clip on your Step-Counter and get moving!

CHAPTER SIX

START LOSING

Cutting Your Calories, Increasing Your Nutrients, Balancing Your Energy

If you think this chapter is about dieting, think again. If you are thinking about crash dieting or joining the latest craze in dieting, we hope you'll rethink that too. Why? Because, quite simply, diets don't work and they aren't good for you. Study after study confirms the indisputable reality that suddenly and severely slashing calories, restricting any essential food group (like carbs), eating excessive amounts of any food (like grapefruits) or food group (like protein), or limiting yourself to a liquid diet never results in lasting and healthy weight loss. Oh, you might lose weight initially and as long as you're dieting, but as soon as you return to "regular" eating, it all goes to hell in a hand-basket … and the fat straight to your stomach, hips, and thighs. Often, you'll end up heavier and fatter than you were before you started dieting. The only thing these hype-driven dietary "magic formulas" have managed to accomplish is to give rise to a multi-billion-dollar industry of weight loss products, books, magazines, experts, and

> **"One should eat to live,
> not live to eat."**
>
> *—Moliere*

businesses. Unfortunately, the well-intentioned consumers who get sucked into these fad diets—people who sincerely want and often need to lose weight for health reasons—are left holding that heavy bag of excess poundage and carting around all that unhealthy fat.

The reality is that the only effective way to reach and sustain your optimal weight, and consequently to live a longer and healthier life, is to make habitual dietary and activity changes in your lifestyle. That's the honest-to-good-health truth. Just ask Oprah.

Diets are a short-term change. Adopting better eating habits is a long-term change. Eating for lasting health is a lifelong change. To lose fat and keep it off, you need to balance your caloric intake with your energy output, by systematically cutting calories, cutting back on unhealthy foods, and adding healthy foods to your "normal" everyday diet 80 to 90 percent of the time. You read that correctly. You don't need to eat perfectly 100 percent of the time. In fact, it is ridiculous to think that anyone could possibly eat a totally balanced and healthy diet every day of their lives and never allow themselves any indulgences. Graduations, birthdays, holidays, and barbecues happen, and food is an important part of celebrations in every society and culture.

With that in mind, no foods are completely off-limits with the 10,000-Steps-A-Day Program. Instead, we recommend limiting "not-so-good foods" and getting sufficient "good foods" on a regular (80-90%) basis. Also, if one of your goals is to lose weight, you'll need to reduce your calories—slowly, sensibly, and safely—and then try to maintain a balance of calories consumed to calories used.

Food Is Fuel

The body uses fuel (food and water) to function in much the same way that a car uses fuel (gas, oil, transmission fluid, coolant, water) to operate. Our digestive system (primarily the stomach, liver, and small intestine) works in concert with our central nervous (brain) and endocrine system (thyroid and adrenal) to convert food to fuel and then to direct that fuel to perform the body's myriad operations. Like vehicles, some bodies run more efficiently than others, due to a host of contributing factors, ranging from age and model (body type) to manufacturer (genetics), maintenance, and usage (exercise). Regardless of those factors, if you don't give your body the proper amounts of the right fuels, you can count on it running poorly, breaking down, and eventually conking out.

In order to perform any activity—whether it's pressing the buttons on the remote control or walking around the block—a chain of complex fuel-driven events must take place within your body.

One of the first links in that chain of events is that the brain sends signals to the appropriate muscles, instructing them to contract. The body uses fuel in the form of glucose to help generate the transmission of these signals. The signals are received by myofilaments, the smallest units of muscle, which release a biochemical called adenosine triphosphate (ATP), which stimulates the muscle to contract, creating movement.

Each time the brain signals a muscle to move, several molecules of ATP must be present in order to fuel the muscle contraction. No ATP, no muscle movement. Not enough ATP, insufficient muscle movement.

Here's the glitch: Our muscles never contain more than a very small amount of ATP. In fact, at any given time you have only enough ATP to run all-out for a little more than 10 seconds. Fortunately, the human body has adapted a work-around to this dilemma: It continuously "recycles" the small amount of ATP we do have by making use of three "fuels" that are present in large amounts through the foods we eat.

These fuels are better known as fat, carbohydrate, and protein. Each of these food fuels allows the body to recycle ATP at different rates and at varying degrees of efficiency, depending on how intensely your body is working. Knowing a little about how these fuels function can help you to hone in on:

Start Losing Some Fuels

You can get started on the road to your optimal weight right now—today—without knowing one other thing about nutrition, without planning a healthier menu, and without restocking your kitchen. Though all those things, in combination with exercise, will definitely help you to lose weight, you can kick-start your weight management program immediately by simply cutting 100 calories a day. Just like with steps, it all adds up. And in this case, less is mo' better.

Here are just a few of the hundreds of ways you can put 100 fewer calories into your body:

- Have a smaller glass of juice (3-4 oz.) and a smaller bowl for cereal (1 cup).
- Substitute a glass of nonfat or 1% milk for milk with a higher fat content.
- Split a bagel with someone, or save half for an afternoon snack or for tomorrow.
- Skip the yolks and eat only egg whites. Another option: if you eat more than one egg for breakfast (however cooked), skip the yolk for at least one of the eggs.
- Order a small soft taco (6 to 8-inch) rather than the larger burrito.
- Skip the croutons on your salad.
- Grill your sandwich using nonstick cooking spray instead of butter.
- Use tuna packed in water rather than oil.
- Reduce your portion of pasta, potatoes, or rice by half a cup.
- Use one pat (1 tablespoon) less of butter or margarine on vegetables, potatoes, bread.
- Limit meat portions to 3 to 4 ounces.
- Leave 3 or 4 bites on your plate.
- Have one dip of ice cream rather than a bowlful.
- Choose a slice of fruit pie over pecan or cream pie.
- Select canned fruit packed in its own juices or water rather than in heavy syrup.
- Eat 10 fewer chips or 1 less handful of mixed nuts.

How much of each fuel you need to consume daily
- Which "empty fuels" to avoid
- Which of these fuels work best with exercise to help you lose fat and strengthen muscle

Nutrition 101

Knowledge is power, and without giving you flashbacks to your high school health class, the following is a quick cheat sheet of nutritional items and terms. Yes, you've heard all of this time and again for years. But a quick refresher won't hurt and could help you to better manage your weight. Don't worry, you won't be tested.

Calories. A calorie is simply a unit of energy. It is the fuel your body burns to do even the slightest task. Calories come from protein, carbohydrates, or fat. The problem comes from over-fueling our bodies—ingesting way more calories than we need.

Smart Choice: Burn more calories than you eat.

Protein. Made up of several different amino acids, protein is the raw material your body uses to make muscle, hair, nails, and skin. Dietary protein contains 4 calories per gram. It keeps you full longer and can help stabilize blood sugar levels.

Smart Choices: Chicken breast, turkey, fish (tuna, sea bass, snapper and many others), nonfat milk, nonfat cottage cheese, lean cuts of beef (sirloin, top round, flank steak), shrimp, soybeans, and protein smoothies.

Carbohydrates. The main source of energy for your body, carbs are the fuel you burn while exercising. Carbs, like protein, contain 4 calories per gram. Sugar is a "simple carb." "Complex carbs," such as whole grains, are a healthier choice.

Smart Choices: Whole grains, whole-wheat bread, sweet potatoes, vegetables, fruits, and oatmeal

Fiber. Designated as a carbohydrate, fiber is actually the indigestible part of plant matter. Fiber is vitally important for optimal digestion and elimination of wastes. It also helps lower cholesterol, decrease certain cancer risks (such as colorectal cancer), and can even help you lose fat by speeding foods through your gut before their fat content is absorbed.

Smart Choices: Beans, some cereals, oatmeal, vegetables (broccoli, spinach, leafy greens, Brussels sprouts), fruit (strawberries, blueberries, raspberries, apples, oranges), and whole grains, such as whole wheat and oat bran

Fat. Although fat contains 9 calories per gram, more than twice the load of carbs and proteins, it is not wise or healthy to eliminate it from your diet. Fat is necessary for hormone production and helps you feel full; healthy fats even help you burn body fat. The trick is choosing the good fats over the not-so-good ones.

Smart Choices: Salmon, mackerel, olive oil, avocados, nuts, seeds, and natural nut butters

Water. The most important nutrient of all, water is constantly overlooked as part of a healthy diet. Like oil in an engine, water is essential for all bodily processes, from digestion to temperature regulation. Focus on nonalcoholic, non-caffeinated beverages.

Smart Choices: Water, sparkling water, unsweetened iced tea, low-calorie sports waters (such as Propel), vegetable juices, clear soups, green tea, herbal teas, and limited amounts of 100% fruit juice (which can be high in sugar, so watch the calories)

Eat to Lose

By now, we all know that the only way to shed pounds and keep them off is to exercise regularly, reduce calories, cut back on calorie-rich foods, such as butter, oils, red meat, full-fat cheeses, and desserts, and cut way back (if not out) nutrient-poor foods such as processed anything. But making relatively simple changes in your daily eating habits can go a long way in helping to rev up your metabolism and burn even more calories. Here are five of the smartest weight-loss life strategies you can make now:

1. Eat breakfast. Turns out, your mom was right: It is bad to skip breakfast. Studies show that skipping breakfast increases the risk of obesity (one more piece of evidence that skipping meals does not

help you lose weight), decreases mental alertness, and is associated with such unhealthy behaviors as smoking, junk-food snacking, and lack of exercise. Yet, how many times do you dash head-first into your day or out the door to work with nothing but coffee in your stomach? By 10:00 A.M., you're hungry and grumpy, and if someone were to offer you a doughnut, you'd gobble it (or two or three) up like you hadn't eaten all day. Small wonder, since you haven't eaten since yesterday, at least 8 hours ago. When you wake up in the morning, your body has already been without food for eight hours, probably more, depending on how long it's been since you ate the evening before.

Eating breakfast makes it easier to resist temptation. To put the final kibosh on sweet but empty temptations, eat a balanced breakfast that includes complex carbohydrates and a little fat, such as egg whites, turkey bacon, or yogurt. Protein helps you feel full longer.

2. Eat smaller amounts more often. "Grazing" is one of the most important fat-loss habits you can pick up. Eating smaller meals more frequently, rather than cramming all your daily calories into two or three squares, helps stave off hunger pangs during the day, which can make you reach for an unhealthy snack in an attempt to give your flagging body a boost in energy. Also, small meals do not initiate certain triggers in your body that tell it to store fat in the

way larger meals do, and grazing won't leave you feeling sluggish the way "gorging" (very large, heavy meals) does.

3. Keep healthy "small meals," like ready-to-drink shakes or a small bowl of cereal, and healthy snacks, such as protein bars and carrot sticks, on hand. Fruits, nuts, cottage cheese, canned tuna, soybeans, turkey jerky, or even half a turkey sandwich are great grazing foods. Make sure to eat all of your smaller meals (or three squares and in-between meal snacks) at about the same time every day. Studies show that eating irregularly can slow metabolism, reduce the "thermic effect" of food (calories burned in processing food), and is linked with obesity and diabetes.

4. Eat more early and less later. For many people, the daily eating ritual goes like this: a cup of coffee and muffin in the morning, a hasty lunch, and then hours later a huge dinner followed by dessert and non-stop snacking until just a few minutes before bed. If you look at calories as fuel and the way in which our bodies naturally use fuel, we have it backwards. We are starving ourselves during the most active part of our day and nutritionally gearing up to run a marathon right before we hit the sack. A smarter idea is to pyramid your food intake. Have a bigger breakfast, a mid-morning snack, and a satisfying lunch. Then have a light afternoon snack and a modest dinner. Your final larger meal should come around three hours before bedtime. A small snack before bedtime is fine.

The Truth about Carbs

Carbohydrates have gotten a bad rap over the years; sometimes for legitimate reasons but mainly for the wrong reasons. The prevalent misconception has been that carbohydrates are bad because they always convert immediately to stored fat. Although carbs do convert to fat when we eat too much or exercise too little (or more likely both), the other important truth about carbs is that they are a vital source of fuel for physical activity.

Our muscles perform very efficiently when burning carbs at all levels of activity, from very low-level aerobic exercise to the most intense anaerobic workouts. Carbohydrate is so critical to muscular functioning that when muscles run out of their stored form of carbohydrate, muscular work ceases completely. In fact, this is what happens when top athletes "hit the wall."

The carbohydrates in the food we eat are broken down primarily by the stomach and liver and converted to glucose. A portion of the glucose is used immediately by the brain, for basic bodily functions, and by activated muscles. Some excess carbohydrate can be stored as glycogen in the muscles and the liver for later use. Because our bodies can store only very limited amounts of glycogen and because we tap into this glycogen supply so often during the day, regular carbohydrate consumption is vital to physical performance.

However, once these glycogen storage areas are full (and these reserve tanks don't hold much), most of the remaining carbohydrate gets converted to fat. Total carbohydrate storage capacity in the liver and muscles ranges from just 200 to 500 grams (about 800 to 2,000 calories' worth) of glycogen.

Under ideal conditions, active individuals would eat small amounts of carbohydrate throughout the day, "grazing" just enough to provide a constant supply of this muscle fuel to give us a steady level of energy without tapping into our glycogen reserves, altering our blood glucose levels, or causing us to store any excess carbohydrate as fat. In reality, because most of us eat once only every several hours, what often happens is that we "gorge" ourselves on carbohydrates. This can start a cascade of undesirable events that leads to low energy and more stored fat.

One of the keys to maintaining a steady flow of carbohydrate is to consume most of your carbs in the form of complex carbohydrates and to limit the amount of simple carbohydrates (sugars) in your diet. Complex carbohydrates are foods that contain long chains of sugars that take a while to break down in the stomach and are released slowly and steadily into the bloodstream, supplying a more uniform level of blood glucose over time. This reduces the amount of insulin released by the pancreas, which in turn reduces the amount of glucose that gets converted into fat and stored in the fat cells.

On the other hand, simple sugars—like those found in many processed foods, breakfast cereals, desserts, and other sweets—break down very rapidly. Although this process can be favorable under certain limited circumstances (like when you are 50 miles into a heavy-duty mountain bike ride or 2 hours into a marathon run, and your glycogen reserves are completely depleted), the more usual result of eating simple sugars is that we store whatever we do not immediately burn off as fat.

The other key to smart carb consumption is to spread it out over the day, avoiding single large carbohydrate meals in favor of smaller and more frequent meals or snacks. There is also some scientific evidence indicating that it is beneficial to "stack" your carbs so that you eat the most in the morning and reduce the amount you consume with each meal.

Bottom line: Carbs are an essential and high-octane fuel for your body, but they give low mileage and have limited storage capacity. So, if you consistently take in more carbs than you can burn off relatively quickly, excess carbs can cause you to gain weight and prevent you from losing it. If you exercise regularly, eat a balanced diet, and avoid simply sugars, carbs are not only okay, they're good for you.

Since carbohydrates are the main food source for energy and since people tend to be more sedentary and burn fewer calories in the evening, it is also a good strategy is to consume the majority of your carbs early in the day and to stick with protein and vegetables in the late afternoon and early evening.

5. Eat whole foods. Try to choose foods that are as close to their natural state and as "close to the farm" as possible. Whenever possible, choose fresh or frozen, and organic if you can and can afford

it. Try not to eat packaged foods, and choose glass and paper packaging over plastic and tin cans. Processed foods tend to be low on nutrients and high on preservatives, including sodium (salt), and other chemicals. The cooking involved in processing tends to rob food of its nutrients and change its natural properties. Many of the important cancer-fighting substances found in fresh produce—nutrients called phytochemicals—are missing in most pre-packaged fare. Often, food that has been processed has been stripped of its fiber, which the body needs for digestion. Plus, many processed foods have high amounts of a synthetic form of "bad" fat, called trans fat, which is even worse for you than the saturated fat found in butter, steak, and whole milk.

In addition to the incredible nutritional value of whole foods, they also have fewer calories. They are also packed with fiber and water, which help you get full faster and feel full longer, and give a greater sense of satisfaction from eating, often referred to as "satiation." So, instead of hitting the drive-by for a "hot apple pie," try reaching for a real apple.

6. Eat, don't drink, your calories. Americans are getting more of their daily calories from the beverages they drink. At the same time, the consumption of nutritious drinks, such as fruit juices and milk, are dwindling while consumption of sugar-laden beverages, like soda, is steadily rising. Meanwhile, as we're guzzling more calo-

True or False: Eating After Dark Is a Big Fat No-No False ... but

with a few conditions. Numerous studies have found no link between when you eat and whether you put on weight, and no scientific evidence that eating late in the evening or just before bed has an effect on weight gain. A 2005 study found that eating late at night has no effect on weight gain even among people with "night eating syndrome" (wake during the night to eat). Another recent study found that women who ate more than 52% of their calories after 5:00 P.M. and who ate after 8:00 P.M. were no more likely to gain weight than those who did not.

That said, people who overeat in general tend to overeat at night (and, for some, during the night), and they tend to eat more calorie-rich foods, both day and night. Naturally, these chronic overeaters are usually overweight or obese.

Evening snacking can put even people who normally eat a balanced diet over their daily calorie quota. Once they've eaten their last large meal, many, if not most, people have reached (or surpassed) the amount of calories their bodies can burn that day, so adding an after-dinner or bedtime snack is simply adding excess calories.

It's not eating at night that makes you gain weight. It's eating too much during the course of the entire day—morning, noon, and night combined—that causes your body to store the excess calories as fat. Weight gain results from a chronic energy imbalance, when total calorie intake exceeds total calorie utilization continuously, week after week and month after month—not hour by hour.

So, you can feel free to eat whenever you want to eat ... as long as the total calories you consume most days doesn't exceed the total calories you burn most days.

True or False (Continued)...

It's also wise to moderate what you eat throughout the day, selecting lighter nutrient-dense over heavier calorie-rich foods, especially at night. Richer foods are often more difficult to digest, and indigestion can interfere with sleep, and not getting enough sleep can slow down the body's metabolism, and a reduced metabolism leads to increased weight. (See how it's all connected?) Alcohol and caffeine have a similar effect on sleep, with similar effects on metabolism and weight gain.

>>tip
Natural Order

Generally, the fewer legs an animal has, the better it is for you. Fish is better than chicken or turkey. Poultry is better than beef or pork. This isn't an absolute—for example, grilled pork loin has less fat than a fried chicken thigh—but it's an easy rule of thumb to remember.

ries and getting fewer nutrients from them, we're also eating as much food (if not more) than ever—a double whammy to our health. So, save most of your calories for food and replace unhealthy drinks with nutritious ones, like low-fat milk, 100% fruit juices, and that good old refreshing, calorie-free, essential liquid, H20.

How Much Is Too Much?

One of the most difficult aspects of weight management is figuring out how many calories you need each day in order to lose weight, sustain your weight, or gain weight. One of the reasons estimating one's personal daily calorie needs is so difficult is because every body is different. Another is because not only does it vary from one person to another, it can also vary for a single person from day to day. For that reason and others, it is important to consult with your doctor if you have a medical condition, are severely overweight, or have been inactive for 6 or more months. Otherwise, though talking with a physician or registered dietitian can be helpful, it is not essential.

In order to determine how many calories to try to shave from each day, you need to have some idea of how many calories you currently consume. The following formula will give you a ballpark of how many calories and grams of fat you need to sustain your current weight.

1. Multiply your body weight by the standard calorie-per-pound for your gender and activity level.

FitnessFACT
Early to Satiate, Early to Lose

An experiment conducted by the Department of Psychology at the University of Texas, El Paso, found that the participants who ate large breakfasts tended to eat fewer calories as the day progresses. Inversely, those who ate large evening meals had a higher rate of caloric intake throughout the day. Those who ate their larger meals earlier in the day also reported experiencing greater satisfaction from their food than those who saved their largest meal for dinner. So, not only does stacking your calories in the early hours keep your body from storing fat, it can also encourage you to eat fewer calories throughout the day.

Moderately Active Male

    ___ pounds x 15 calories = ___ total calories per day

Moderately Active Female

    ___ pounds x 12 calories = ___ total calories per day

Relatively Active Male

    ___ pounds x 13 calories = ___ total calories per day

Relatively Active Female

    ___ pounds x 10 calories = total calories per day

2. Multiply your total calories per day by 30 percent.

    ___ calories per day x .30 = ___ calories from fat per day

3. Divide your total grams of fat per day by 9 (the number of calories per gram).

    ___ calories from fat per day ÷ 9 = ___ fat grams per day

If you want to lose weight, you will need to reduce your daily intake of calories and fat by whatever amount exceeds the amounts indicated above (give or take a few hundred calories to account for differences among people). The first place to start cutting calories

>>**tip**
Stop the Pop

We can't Splenda®-coat this: Stop drinking soda immediately. You will see amazing results from this one simple change. In fact, if you normally drink two sodas a day and you give them up, you can lose 10 pounds in a year without making any other changes. If you drink more soda than that and give it all up, you can lose even more.

is with things you eat and drink that are not essential to your health (see "Making Healthy Food Choices, below) and that impede your health.

Making Healthy Food Choices

In 2005, the USDA replaced the old "meat-and-potatoes" heavy dietary guidelines with a new "Food Pyramid" that is based on years of comprehensive scientific research. The guidelines outline a "healthy diet," not a therapeutic one, for "the general public" over the age of 2 years, and suggest that anyone with specific health concerns consult their doctors regarding their individual dietary needs and restrictions. The 2005 Dietary Guidelines for Americans defines "healthy diet" as one that includes:

- Fruits and vegetables
- Lean protein (meats, poultry, fish, eggs, nuts, beans)
- Whole grains (at least half of daily allowance)
- Fat-free or low-fat sources of calcium (milk and milk products)
- Low amounts of saturated fats, trans fats, cholesterol, salt (sodium), and added sugars

• Allows for a limited amount of "discretionary" (you choose) food choices, in addition to the daily recom mended amounts of each food group

Of course, not even Uncle Sam can tell you exactly what quantity of each food group and which specific foods within each group are best for you. That depends (like everything else related to human physiology) on myriad individual factors, including age, gender, level of activity, genetics, any health conditions you might have, and any medications you might be taking—not to mention your own likes and dislikes. Food, like exercise, is a very personal thing. But the following are good general guidelines for adults who get in about 30 minutes of daily exercise:

Is Meat Protein Better than Plant Protein?

Many people are under the impression that protein from meat is of a higher quality than protein from plant sources. It is not. Amino acids are amino acids, whether they come from plants or animals. The real question is whether you are getting all of the amino acids you need in your diet. Although humans are able to recycle many of the 22 amino acids that comprise protein, our bodies are unable to manufacture 8 of them. These 8 amino acids have become known as "essential" amino acids, because getting them in our diet is essential to health. Whereas most animal protein contains all 22 amino acids in various amounts, most plant sources do not, and the configuration and amount of the amino acids in plants varies greatly. Still, within the plant kingdom, all 22 amino acids can be accounted for quite easily by combining different grains, fruits, and vegetables. As long as you are getting all 22 amino acids from one source or another, in particular the appropriate amounts of the 8 "essential" amino acids, your body won't care whether they come from animal or vegetable sources.

The main benefit to a diet that includes meat, chicken, and fish is that your requirements for complete protein can be met quite easily. The drawback is that animal protein sources also tend to be higher in fat. However, by trimming off visible fat, eliminating skin, broiling instead of frying, and eating smaller portions, you can get ample amounts of protein while minimizing your fat intake.

On the other hand, some people feel that a vegetarian diet not only is a legitimate source of high quality protein but also a healthier alternative, because plant sources are almost always lower in fat—except for certain protein-rich foods like nuts, seeds, avocados, and some types of tofu. Just make certain that you are obtaining your total daily protein requirements and that you are getting all of the essential amino acids. The best way for vegetarians to ensure this is to regularly include beans, lentils, peas, and other legumes in their diets. These supply cer-

>>**tip**

Timeline for Slimmer Lines

For best results—to maximize fat loss and your odds of keeping it off, and to minimize drops in your metabolism and energy—decrease your calorie intake by 300 to 500 calories per day, while simultaneously increasing your physical activity. If you are obese or very overweight, a weight loss of 1 to 2 pounds per week is acceptable. If you have only a few pounds to drop, the rate should not exceed 0.5 to 1 pound per week. Otherwise, a rate of 0.5 to 2 pounds per week is recommended.

tain amino acids absent in grains, fruits, and leafy vegetables, and when the vegetables are eaten in the right amounts and combination, they can provide all your essential amino acids.

Oil Okays and Oil Avoids

Your body needs some fat to function properly. Oils are a form of fat that is liquid at room temperature. Oils are used primarily in cooking (for example, canola, corn, olive, peanut, sunflower) and to a lesser extent as flavoring (walnut, hazelnut, fish, sesame).

Most cooking and flavoring oils come from plants. Vegetable and nut oils contain no cholesterol, and they are typically high in unsaturated fats and low in saturated fat (the not-so-good stuff). However, some plant fats, like coconut and palm oil, are high in saturated fats, and so for dietary purposes should be treated as solid fats. Solid fats include butter, vegetable shortening, stick margarine, lard (pork fat), beef fat (tallow, suet), and chicken fat. All animal fat contains cholesterol.

Fitness FACT
Prevention Is the Best Intention

For most people, it is easier not to gain weight in the first place than it is to lose weight once they've packed it on. The more weight you gain, the more difficult it is to take it off. And it only gets more difficult once you hit middle age. So, make not gaining another unwanted pound your goal. Adding just 30 minutes of exercise to your daily routine and eating just 100 fewer calories a day can help you to stop gaining weight.

Many processed foods contain oil, and some—including mayonnaise and some soft margarines and salad dressings, are made mostly of oil. These processed food products are often high in saturated fats and trans fat.

Trans fat, also called trans fatty acids (TFAs), is the result of a process called hydrogenation, which is used to turn liquid fats into solids. Manufacturers use hydrogenation because foods that contain hydrogenated oils have a longer shelf life and retain a moist and delicious mouthfeel. However, trans fats have significant health consequences, such as increasing the bad form of cholesterol, clogging arteries, and contributing to adult-onset diabetes. As of January 2006, food companies are now required to list the trans fat content of their foods. Read the labels, and avoid packaged cookies and crackers, margarine, doughnuts, fried foods, and anything that contains the words "hydrogenated vegetable oils" in the ingredient list.

Of these oils, unsaturated fat is the most beneficial and least harmful to your body, while too much saturated fat can negatively

Daily Recommended Food Allowances

Gender	Age	Veggies	Fruit	Grains	Meats/Beans	Milk	Oils
Women							
	19-30	2 cups	2 cups	3 ounces	5 ounces	3	6 teaspoons
	31-50	2 cups	1 cups	3 ounces	5 ounces	3	5 teaspoons
	51-plus	2 cups	1 cups	3 ounces	5 ounces	3	5 teaspoons
Men							
	19-30	3 cups	2 cups	4 ounces	6 ounces	3	7 teaspoons
	31-50	3 cups	2 cups	3 ounces	6 ounces	3	6 teaspoons
	51-plus	2 cups	2 cups	3 ounces	5 ounces	3	6 teaspoons

impact your health. With saturated fats, less is always better. With unsaturated fats, you can't go wrong with that age-old advice: "Moderation in all things." Trans fat is just plain bad in any amount and should be avoided.

Reading Food Labels

You can eat a healthy diet and lose weight as long as you pay attention to what you're eating. Reading and knowing how to interpret food labels will give you a leg up in that regard, at least in terms of packaged food.

As of 1994, all packaged food must include a label citing nutritional information that conforms to standards established by the Food and Drug Administration. Reading the "nutrition fact" label

FitnessFACT
Shake the Salt Habit

is the easiest way to get a handle on exactly what's in the food you are eating. These newer labels have fairly realistic estimations of "serving size." Regardless of whether you consider the portion or serving amount appropriate for you, keep in mind that the rest of the label contains information relative only to this listed serving size or portion, and not necessarily to the whole container's worth of food.

Therefore, if you intend to eat double or triple (or half) the listed serving size, make sure to double or triple (or halve) all the other numbers on the label.

Following are explanations of a few of the more important labeling terms:

Calories per Serving. The number of calories for the recommended serving. If your serving is larger or smaller, your calories will be more or fewer.

Over time, the American palate has grown accustomed to the flavor that salt brings to food, and we generally eat far too much of it for our own good. Medical research has shown that excessive salt can cause or increase the risk of high blood pressure and strokes. Also, salt causes fluid retention, and "bloating" is definitely not a "lean" quality.

As a rule of thumb, you should restrict your salt intake to under 2,000 mg (about 1 teaspoon) of salt per day. Even if you don't use a salt shaker, you should still pay attention to how much salt you're getting through "hidden" sources, such as packaged and restaurant foods. Remember, mustard, catsup, pickles, salad dressings, cereals, snacks, packaged nuts, canned soups, and meat jerky can be high in sodium. Read labels and police your salt intake.

Fitness FACT
Number One Source of Fat for Women

Chocolate? Pastries? Cookies? Potato chips? Ice cream? Butter? Meat? Nope. None of those usual suspects. Though many women do get much of their intake of fat with these foods, the culprit at the top of the most-wanted for most-fat-eaten list (at 9% of total fat intake) is salad dressing. Even many "light" dressings contain 40 to 50 calories per tablespoon. While men might not get the bulk of their fat from salad dressing, it's no less fattening for them.

So, read the label and choose the dressing with the least fat and the least amount of saturated fat, and if it has any trans fat, just don't do it. Take your dressing on the side, rather than smothering your salad with it, and dip your greens or drizzle a small amount on them as you eat. Better, go for balsamic vinegar mixed with herbs and a teensy-tiny bit of extra virgin olive oil and no added salt or sugar. Even better, try a squeeze of fresh lemon juice and a light sprinkling of salt and pepper.

Calories from Fat. More important than calories per serving, given the health deficits that come from excess fat. To determine exactly how "fat-free" or fat-laden each serving is, divide "calories from fat" by total calories per serving and multiply by 100 to get "percent calories from fat." If it is less than 30%, you should be okay, provided you are eating substantial amounts of complex carbohydrate-rich foods (which will, almost by definition, be very low in fat). Even if the food in question contains fat in an amount higher than 30%, your main goal number is still total fat grams per day.

% Daily Value. A general reference guide based on an assumed daily caloric intake of 2,000 and the government's recommendation that 30% of your calories come from fat and 60% from carbs. Keep in mind that you daily calorie goal is not necessarily that recommended by the USDA; we encourage you to determine your own optimal calories-per-day and fat-per-calories-per-day, consulting with a doctor of dietician, as needed.

Obviously, the big number everyone is concerned with is fat, and all labels get this news out of the way first. Total fat grams (per serving) is what we are most interested in tracking, so pay close attention to this one. As for the saturated/unsaturated breakdown, as mentioned before, if your total fat intake is under control and you are eating mostly unprocessed foods, you should be okay.

Total Carbohydrate. The main number to seek out in this category. Higher dietary fiber is considered good; a low number for "Sugar" is also considered good, because this refers to simple sugars. Assume that most of whatever is not sugars will be complex carbs. Remember that we are looking to get a handle on grams per day.

Protein per Serving. This ought to be self-explanatory. Remember, though, this won't identify the amino acid breakdown of your protein, just total grams per day.

Vitamins. Vitamin and mineral content is expressed only as a percent of the government's recommended daily dosage (RDA).

Hydration

Water is essential for human life. Over 70% of the human body consists of water; muscles actually have a higher percentage and are close to 85% water. Virtually all chemical reactions that occur in the body require water. Without water, the human body can sustain life for only a few days. When exercising, the body depends on water to cool itself (through sweat) and to help eliminate toxins. Water helps us metabolize fats easier.

Clearly, adequate water intake is an important part of any nutrition and exercise program. Most experts advise drinking the equivalent of eight (or more) 8-ounce glasses of water a day. Fortunately, much of the food we eat, especially fruits and vegetables, is high in water content, so if you're not wild for water, you don't necessarily need to walk around with a bottle in your hands all day. Juices, teas, soups, and other forms of liquid (except alcohol) count also.

Still, no liquid is better for your body than water, and everybody needs to drink several glasses of water a day—in addition to the water they get from other foods and beverages—to keep your body healthy and running smoothly. So, pay attention to the amount of water you are drinking and make an effort to take in at least eight cups of water (or substitute a few of those cups with a healthy equivalent) every day.

Dehydration

When your body uses and excretes (sweat, urine) more fluid than it takes in, the amount of water remaining in the body drops below the level it needs to operate efficiently. Small and temporary decreases are no cause for alarm, and most people are unaware of minor levels of dehydration. But larger levels and longer durations of dehydration, which will make you feel lousy and zap your energy and can have serious harmful effects. And by the time you feel the ill effects of dehydration, your body is long past the point of adequate hydration.

Not drinking enough water and other healthy fluids is the most common cause of low to moderate levels of dehydration. Having a gastrointestinal illness, like the stomach flu, or a hangover—anything that causes vomiting and/or diarrhea—can also cause dehydration. So can using diuretics (coffee, tea, diet pills) and spending too much time in the sauna, Jacuzzi, steamy shower, or hot bath water.

Your body generally needs more water during hot weather (3 to 4 quarts, and up to 3 gallons a day) and when you exercise regularly. Your body always uses more water more quickly during intense workouts, and so it is important to drink extra fluids before, during, and after the activity. As a rule of thumb: drink 1/2-1 cup of water for every 15 to 20 minutes of exercise.

Chronic dehydration poses serious health risks. For example, it can cause abnormal potassium and salt levels in the body, which can lead to irregular heart rhythms. Chronic dehydration can also be a sign of a serious underlying health problem, such as diabetes. If you are often dehydrated, you should consult with your physician.

Whether you feel dehydrated often, sometimes, or never, you should always make it a point to drink your daily recommended allowance of water (64 ounces), drink more when your body heats up (whether through exercise, hot showers, or hot weather), and avoid diuretics.

Food Fit for Exercise

How much you eat and how soon you eat before and after exercising can affect your physical performance. Your food choices can also help or hinder your workout.

Exercising too soon after a large meal can make you feel sluggish and nauseous, and it can cause stomach and muscle cramping, even diarrhea. That's because your body is trying to do things that require energy and blood supply at the same time: digest your food and provide fuel to your muscles.

On the other hand, exercising when you haven't given your body enough of the right fuels before the activity can result in too-low blood sugar levels. Then, you're apt to feel weak and tired and to be less alert and coordinated. Consequently, you will probably cut back on both the duration and intensity of your workout. It also increases your risk of injury.

Timed to Exercise

To time your eating for maximum exercise results:
- Eat a full breakfast that includes both complex carbohydrates and protein.
- Eat larger meals 3 to 4 hours before exercising.
- Eat smaller meals 2 or 3 hours before exercising.
- Eat a light, nutrition-dense snack 5 to 15 minutes before exercise or during long walks/hikes. Ideal: carbs + protein, 200-300 calories.
- Eat within 2 hours after exercising.
- Don't skip meals.

Best Foods for Peak Performance

To provide optimal fuel for your exercise, eat the right types and amounts of these foods:

Carbohydrates. Your body stores carbs as glycogen, which your muscles rely on for energy. A diet containing 40 to 50% of calories from complex carbohydrates is recommended for most people; people in excellent physical condition with low body fat who exercise often and intensely may require more. Good carbs for exercise: vegetables, fruit, rice, and whole-grain breads and cereals. Avoid eating fruit and high-fiber foods (beans, lentils, bran cereals) just before an intense workout. Fructose, a simple sugar found in fruit, when combined with heavy exercise, can increase the risk of diarrhea; similarly, high-fiber foods can cause excess gas and cramping.

Protein and fats. Although protein is not the ideal source for fueling muscles, it plays an important role in muscle repair and growth. Most people get enough protein in their normal diets and do not need additional protein supplements. Avoid eating foods with high fat contents before exercising; fat takes longer to digest and can make you feel uncomfortable. Good proteins and fats for exercise: Lean meat, low-fat or nonfat dairy products (milk, cottage cheese, yogurt, natural white cheeses), nuts, fish, vegetable oils (olive, canola, sunflower).

Food and Sleep: The Weight-Loss Connection

When you get the munchies, it's not always because you're hungry; sometimes it's because you're tired. People who are sleep-deprived have decreased levels of a hormone that regulates appetite, called leptin. Studies have shown that when people don't get enough zzz's, they feel hungrier and tend to eat more, increasing their risk of weight gain. People who get enough sleep

Nutritional Supplements

In an era of heavily processed foods and nutrient-depleted soils, covering your nutritional bases with a little supplemental help can be a good idea. All of the following are found in whole foods, but would be difficult to get enough of with even a perfect diet. Remember, people who exercise regularly have greater nutritional requirements than those who do not. The daily recommended dosages listed are for adults. Depending on your age and gender, you might require higher or lesser amounts and additional nutrients.

Supplement	Daily Recommended Dosage	Benefit
Vitamin E	400–800 IU	Antioxidant, helps reduce exercise-related muscle damage, especially for people just starting a workout program.
Vitamin C	250–500 mg	Enhances the function of your immune system, reduces post-workout inflammation, improves joint health, fight cancer-causing free radicals.
Multivitamin	1 serving after breakfast vitamin or mineral deficiencies.	Improve overall health and prevent
Calcium	1,200 mg helps burn fat.	Essential for bone health as well as for neuro-muscular impulses during exercise; research suggests dairy-source calcium (low-fat yogurt and skim milk)
Essential Fatty Acids	1 tablespoon	Boosts overall health, improves heart health, optimizes key hormones, even aids in fat loss.

are less hungry and eat less, decreasing their risk of weight gain.

Most people need 7 to 8 hours of sleep a night. If something disturbs your sleep and you're feeling tired the next day, be aware that those "hunger pangs" you're feeling might be your sleep-deprived body's way of telling you that you need more rest, not more calories. Rather than give in to that late afternoon sugar fix you might be craving (another hallmark of exhaustion-related hunger), try taking a 15-minute nap or rest period … and then eat a light snack of 200 to 300 calories that includes a complex carbohydrate (no sugary stuff) and protein.

When and what you eat throughout the day and particularly in the hours before you normally go to sleep can have an effect on how easily you fall asleep and how well you sleep.

>>**tip**

Green Tea Packs a Punch

One cup of green tea before exercise can help increase energy and boost your metabolism to allow for greater fat loss. It also enhances your immune system and helps fight some cancers.

Sleep Aid

Eating a light snack of about 200 calories stimulates the production of serotonin, a hormone that regulates mood. When you have a small bedtime snack of mostly complex carbohydrate (no processed sugars) and a small amount of protein, which contains the "sleepy" amino acid tryptophan (especially prevalent in turkey), the brain produces serotonin, which has a calming effect.

And so you fall asleep more easily and are more lightly to sleep well through the night.

Sleep Stealers

For a good night's sleep, it's best to avoid these foods:

Caffeine: within 3-8 hours before bedtime, in all its lovely liquid and solid forms: coffee, tea, cola drink, chocolate

Liquids: any, including water, within 90 minutes before bedtime

Alcohol: limit anytime of the day, avoid within 90 minutes of bedtime

Heavy meals: less than 3 hours before bedtime

Cooking Healthy Meals

In today's jam-packed, fast-paced lifestyles, it is not always convenient to prepare healthy, tasty meals. When it comes to your health and weight loss, though, nothing beats fresh home cooking, which puts you in full control of what you and your loved ones are eating. The following basic guidelines will help you to prepare healthful meals and snacks.

• Cut back on the use of oils, butter, and margarine. Instead of sautéing in oil, use a non-stick pan or non-stick cooking spray and/or use chicken broth as the liquid. Try to break the bread and butter habit. Enjoy the flavor of the bread (whole-grain is best) by itself or dip it into a low-fat vinaigrette infused with tasty herbs. When you can't avoid using oil, choose canola or olive oil and use sparingly.

• Use non-fat mayonnaise as a sandwich spread, or use mustard or

Signs of Dehydration

- Thirst
- Dizziness
- Feeling light-headed
- Dry or sticky mouth
- Fatigue
- Loss of coordination (especially during physical activity)
- Mental confusion
- Irritability
- Dry skin
- Elevated body temperature
- Decreased and/or darker urine production

salsa instead, and for chicken-salad and tuna-salad.

- Use only non-fat (best) or low-fat (1%) dairy products—milk, yogurt, cottage cheese, cream cheese, sour cream. If a sauce requires cream, substitute evaporated non-fat milk with a little flour.
- Explore the world of fresh herbs and spices to add flavor and satisfaction to your cooking. Vinegar is another addition that adds fat-free zest to foods.
- Homemade soups are easy to make, great "comfort food," and fulfilling. Combine any and all vegetables, condiments, legumes and grains for a healthy and hearty meal. Make clear soups, rather than cream based, and eliminate or at least minimize the use of oil when preparing.
- Egg whites are high in protein, naturally fat free, and make wonderful omelets. Avoid yolks at all costs. When baking, add an extra white to compensate for the missing yolk. If you just can't tolerate all-white scrambled eggs, omelets, and frittatas, use two egg whites and one whole egg.

>>**tip**

Nagged by the Need to Nosh?

Don't let emotional, nervous, and habitual eating munch your health away. When you feel the urge to nibble but you really aren't hungry, get up, get out, and take a short walk instead. People have quit smoking by walking when the urge to smoke strikes, and nicotine tends to be a much more difficult an addiction to break than habitual eating is. Of course, smokers can ban cigarettes completely from their lives, and everyone has to eat. But distracting yourself from eating "just because" by taking a walk will help you eat less and burn more. Every little bit helps.

- Steam, bake in natural juices, or grill your chicken, fish, and lean meat without oil. Freely use herbs and spices, lemon or lime to season. Steam your rice and vegetables without butter or oil.
- Use non-fat salad dressings, mustard, lemon juice,vinegar, or salsa to spruce up greens, steamed vegetables, rice, and baked potatoes.
- Keep your meat portions under five ounces. Better yet, use meat as a flavoring for another dish (vegetable or grain dish).
- Remove all skin and visible fat from chicken an meats.

Healthy Meals and Snacks

Whether you choose to eat at home or eat out, the following will provide a range of foods that fit into a healthy menu. We all have different tastes, so improvise and bring your personal creativity to preparing and ordering your food.

All of these meals will vary in their individual breakdown of carbohydrates, protein, and fat content, but don't get hung up in the details; they all fall within the acceptable range for healthy dining. Please take the time to adjust the portions to your personal calorie needs and eat what is appropriate for your body. The objective here is not to dictate a rigid diet; it's to create an eating lifestyle that is best for your health and for managing your weight.

It might take some time and experimentation to create a full menu of the healthy meals and snacks that not only taste great but also make you feel great. But once you do, eating tasty, healthy meals will become second-nature.

Sample Breakfasts

It is best to start your day with a combination of carbohydrate and protein, either in one food dish or in two or three single foods. Fruit is always good, but complement it with some complex carbohydrates or a light protein to avoid a late-morning energy drop. **Following is one week's worth of smart choices:**

1. Hot oatmeal or high-fiber cold cereal, with fruit and non-fat milk. Low calorie sweetener or a little sugar is acceptable.

2. Egg white omelet in a non-stick pan, with any combination of spinach, mushrooms, tomatoes, salsa, and herbs, with dry whole-grain toast or bagel.

3. Fruit bowl (for example, melons, bananas, grapes) topped with

non-fat yogurt or low-fat cottage cheese, with a non-fat muffin.
4. Whole wheat or oatmeal pancakes with fruit syrup and non-fat yogurt.
5. Low-fat granola with non-fat yogurt and fruit.
6. Bagel with low-fat cream cheese and tomatoes or toasted with 100% fruit spread (no sugar added).
7. Fresh fruit smoothie with low-fat cinnamon roll or bagel.

Acceptable beverages include coffee, tea, fresh fruit juice, mixed vegetable juices, non-fat milk, and mineral water.

Sample Lunches

Your mid-day meal is the cornerstone of your daily nutritional intake. For optimal weight loss, it is best to consume the most calories and nutrients during the most active part of the day (between 11:00 A.M. and 3:00 p.m. for most people), when your metabolism is at its highest.

Here are several healthy choices:
1. Tuna sandwich made with non-fat mayonnaise on whole-grain bread, with vegetarian split pea soup and an apple.
2. Grilled chicken breast or turkey burger on a whole-wheat roll with mustard, lettuce, and tomato, with vegetable soup or green salad.

3. Green salad (dilute dressing) with lentil soup and whole-grain bread.

4. Grilled vegetarian burger on a multi-grain bun, with tomato soup (pureed, not creamed).

5. Turkey and low-fat cheese sandwich on whole-grain bread topped with grated carrots, mustard, lettuce, and tomato. Fruit salad with yogurt.

6. Steamed vegetables and brown rice, with salsa, low-sodium soy sauce or lemon. Whole grain toast with sliced tomatoes.

7. Vegetable salad with grilled tuna or chicken in light vinaigrette dressing. Pita bread and an orange.

8. Chicken enchilada made with breast meat, a small, low-fat corn tortilla, and fresh or low-sodium enchilada, with shredded lettuce, chopped tomato. Fresh melon.

9. Grilled or baked fish with grilled vegetables and steamed rice. Season with low-sodium soy sauce or lemon-pepper.

10. Pasta in marinara sauce, with steamed broccoli or green salad and crusty Italian bread.

11. Cheeseless pizza with grilled chicken, onions, and zucchini. Green salad.

12. Vegetarian burrito with low-fat cheese, rice and non-fat refried beans, salsa, and shredded lettuce.

13. Chicken (breast meat) or fish tacos with low-fat sour cream.

FitnessFACT
Walk-a-Bye Baby

One of the best natural defenses against sleep deprivation is regular exercise—as long as it's not too soon before bedtime. Exercising during the day tends to enhance sleep, but exercising within 3 hours of bedtime can rev you up and make it more difficult to sleep. Studies show that exercising 3 to 6 hours before hitting the sack has the most positive effect on falling and staying asleep.

Green salad with fresh salsa. Orange slices.

14. Baked potato with steamed vegetables and salsa. Cup of lentil soup.

15. Minestrone soup, tomato and cucumber salad, and focaccia.

16. Bagel with smoked salmon and tomato, low-fat cream cheese, fresh fruit salad.

17. Fruit plate with low-fat cottage cheese. Whole wheat rolls.

Drink plenty of water throughout the day. Tea, coffee, fruit juices, vegetable juices, and non-fat milk are fine.

Sample Dinners

After a long day, it is best to wind down your system with a lighter meal. Again, if you feel that you need more food, eat larger portions of vegetables or salad. For optimal fitness conditioning, stick to either strictly a protein meal or a carbohydrate meal, to keep the digestive system efficient and swift.

Here are a few healthy, tasty menu options:

1. Grilled or baked fish or shrimp with steamed vegetables.

2. Chicken or tofu and fresh vegetables stir-fry in ginger-soy broth, with steamed rice.

3. Baked potato with mushrooms sautéed in chicken broth and garlic, with steamed vegetables.

4. Green salad with grilled chicken or turkey strips, low-fat cheese, and garbanzo beans in non-fat dressing.

5. Green peppers stuffed with ground lean turkey and rice. Fresh green beans sprinkled with lemon and almond slivers.

6. Chicken marinara with vegetables and salad.

7. Vegetarian chili with whole wheat rolls. Small green salad with nonfat dressing.

8. Legume (or bean) and vegetable soup, with green salad and non-fat dressing.

9. Instead of dessert, choose fresh fruit to satisfy your sweet tooth.

Sample Healthy Snacks

Portion control is important for all your meals, but it is especially critical to healthful snacking. Avoid eating directly from bulk packaging. There are many snack products to available now that are "fat free" and "baked," but don't take their word for it: Read the labels to make sure the processed food doesn't contain high levels of saturated fats or any trans fat (which you should completely eliminate from your diet). Check the label for calorie and fat grams per serving, and make sure to stay within your "discretionary" calorie quota.

Here are several smart snack choices:

1. Protein shake, made with fruit juice and/or a banana, to boost energy in the late morning or afternoon.

2. Air-popped popcorn, with or without seasoning, but with low salt and no added sugar.

3. Rice cakes, available in multiple flavors. Try topped with sliced bananas, sliced tomatoes with a sprinkling of salt and pepper, low-fat cottage cheese, cucumbers with a sprinkle of seasoning.

4. Baked tortilla chips with fresh salsa.

5. Seasonal fresh fruit—apples, blueberries, pears, oranges, bananas, grapes, strawberries, melons, grapes, peaches, apricots, papaya, mango, etc.

6. Fresh vegetables, sliced or cut into bite-size pieces, or whole—carrots, celery, jicama, snap peas, cherry tomatoes, broccoli, etc. Munch as much as you want. Even better: straight from your garden or the farmer's market, and organic.

6. Vegetable juice, fruit juice, or blended fruit-vegetable juices. Make sure it's 100% fruit juice with no sugar added.

7. Non-fat yogurt or cottage cheese with fresh fruit (blueberries, pineapple, peaches, etc.)

8. Fat-free pretzels (low sodium preferable)

>>tip

Three Fat-Busting Foods

1. Carrots. Eating just 2 carrots a day will lower your cholesterol 10 to 20%.
2. Garlic. Helps to lower cholesterol and blood pressure.
3. Grapes. The skin contains an organic chemical compound that helps lower cholesterol.

9. Dried fruit (raisins, cranberry, blueberry, pineapple, apples, banana, etc.). Make sure the banana is dried and not fried; "banana chips" are deep-fried in coconut oil and loaded with calories (150), fat (10 grams), and sugar—as bad, if not worse, than potato chips.

9. Whole-grain bread, rolls, English muffins, or bagels, toasted or plain.

10. Cup of "clear" soup, low or non-fat (split pea, lentil, chicken rice, vegetable, black bean, pureed tomato, carrot, squash, broccoli, etc.). Steer clear of cream-based soups.

11. Corn on the cob. A perfect energy booster, steamed or uncooked, right off the cob.

12. Unsalted nuts and seeds—walnuts, almonds, filberts, cashews, sunflower seeds, edamame (soy nuts), etc. Limit or avoid macadamia nuts, which are high in fat.

13. High-fiber, low-sugar cereal with non-fat milk and low-calorie sweetener

Eating Out: What to Order

We all know that preparing our own food is the best way to assure that we are eating properly. But there are special occasions when going to a restaurant is enjoyable and days when we just don't have the time to shop and prepare meals. Here are a few tips on what to order when you eat out, whether you opt for fast food restaurant or fine dining.

- Deep fried foods are out. Steamed, baked, poached, or grilled are in. Ask if a sautéed item can be cooked in broth rather than oil.

- Try to find "the closest thing to the farm" as possible. Many fast food chains offer salads or even salad bars. Use good judgment in your choices, avoiding the creamy and oily selections. Stick to the fresh, undressed items, and use non-fat dressing or diluted dressings.

- Ask the waiter how certain food items are prepared. A pasta entrée with chicken and asparagus might sound great, but if the menu fails to mention that it is prepared in a heavy cream sauce, it's not a good choice.

- Ask for the chef to prepare your meal in a way that works for you. If you don't see anything on the menu, ask whether they can grill a chicken breast, or make a plate of steamed vegetables with a baked potato or

Eating Out: What to Order (Continued)

rice, or toss some pasta with tomato marinara sauce.

- Ask for all sauces to be "on the side," including your salad dressing. Hold the "special sauce." Salsa, vinegar, and mustards are safe bets to use instead.

- Choose thin-crusted pizza instead of deep dish varieties. Try a cheeseless pizza with an assortment of toppings such as mushrooms, onions, tomatoes, peppers, basil, and chicken.

- Avoid prepared salads, like cole slaw, potato salad, and marinated salads (such as "three-bean"). Opt, instead, for fresh greens and vegetables, and use dressing sparingly or with lemon, herbs, and vinegar for flavor.

- Avoid chicken wings. Skinless, white breast meat is preferred.

- Fish is usually a good choice, but make sure it is grilled and not breaded, battered, or fried or smothered in a cream or buttery sauce. Avoid tartar sauces.

CHAPTER SEVEN

PICK UP THE PACE

90 Days to Your Optimal Weight and Better Health

The Surgeon General's suggestion to add at least 30 minutes of exercise (about 3,000 steps) and to cut at least 100 calories a day is not intended as a quick fix plan or a stop-gap measure. It is a health strategy for life, and its purpose is to help the average U.S. citizen to at least maintain his or her current weight and level of fitness, thereby reducing the risk of chronic disease by at least that margin of improved fitness. If you, like more than two-thirds of American adults, are overweight or obese, this "at least" fitness strategy is unlikely to bring the weight loss and health improvements you need and desire. If you are among the one-third of the population that is at or below your optimal weight, that does not necessarily mean you will remain at that weight or that you are at your optimal level of fitness.

Studies show that the overwhelming majority of us will be overweight for at least some period in the future or will become overweight as time goes on—including about half of those who are not currently overweight. In fact, one study of 4,000 Caucasian adults revealed that 90% of men and 70% of women were or had become overweight over a 30-year span (1971 to 2001). Even more alarming, one in three of the participants in the study (by the National Heart, Lung, and Blood Institute) were obese or became obese during that timeframe.

The risks of going from healthy weight to overweight and from merely overweight to obese are no less in the short run. According to results from the 1999-2002 National Health and Nutrition Examination Survey, 65% of adults (20 and older) are either overweight or obese, and 30% are obese. What is more, one in five women and one in four men who were at a healthy weight when they entered the study were overweight after four years. Of those who were overweight when the study began, almost 20% of the women and over 12% of the men became obese.

Hundreds of scientific studies have also shown that the only way to lose weight and to sustain a healthy weight over the long-term is to adopt a lifelong habit of exercising regularly and of eating a balanced diet routinely. The most effective way to develop new eating and exercising habits is to make incremental changes gradually and to repeat the same changes consciously and continuously over the course of at least six months. The best way to ensure that these new habits

FitnessFACT
Treading All Over the Competition

Trekking on a treadmill burns more calories and increases cardiovascular fitness more effectively than using a stationery bike, stair-climbers, rowers, and ski machines, according to a study by the Medical College of Wisconsin and the Veterans Affairs Medical Center in Milwaukee.

stick and become lifelong habits is to continue your nutrition and exercise programs for at least a year, until they become routine. Then, to maximize your chances of staying on track and fit for life, it is wise to extend these eating and exercise habits throughout your life, periodically taking stock to modify your nutrition and exercise goals and activities to fit inevitable changes in your life, your body, and your interests.

To help you succeed in reaching and sustaining your fitness goals, the 10,000-Steps-A-Day Program is a six-month program consisting of two 90-day segments. Level One is designed to help you reach the equivalent of the Surgeon General's suggestion to add 30 minutes of daily exercise, or whatever personal goal you've set for yourself. Level Two is designed to help you move toward the optimal goal of 10,000 steps a day (or your personal goal). This chapter focuses on Level Two—on how to add more steps to your day. Later, in Chapter 11, we'll talk about how to step it up even more with a "10,000-Steps-Plus" plan for increasing your steps to 12,000 to 15,000 per day, the amount of physical activity typically needed to lose weight and trim fat.

Fitness**FACT**

City Striders

The wholesome lifestyle of small-town living and the evils of the big city may be more mythology than fact when it comes to exercise. A study in the journal Medicine & Science in Sports & Exercise measured leisure-time physical activity and found that people in large cities had the highest rates of daily activity. Rural residents (especially in the South) had the highest prevalence of inactivity and lowest fitness levels. Score one for the concrete jungle.

Taking It to the Next Level

After 90 days of walking regularly and routinely cutting 100 calories here and 100 calories there, you will no doubt feel better and probably also look trimmer. You might have even lost a few pounds. Those gains are great rewards in and of themselves. But reward can be a great motivator, so upon completing Level One of your 10,000-Steps-A-Day Program, treat yourself to something special—a new outfit or CD, a movie date (hold the butter on the popcorn), a walking tour of a fun city, an afternoon tea (green) with your friends, or dinner out in a favorite restaurant (just watch the fat, calories, and your portions).

At that point, you should also take time to assess your progress and to re-evaluate your goals. Some questions to consider:

• Did you reach or come close to, or fall short of, or exceed your end goal?

• Did you make steady progress, or was your progress irregular?

• Did you set your daily step goals too high or too low or just about right?

- Were your incremental goals (increments of one week, two weeks, three weeks, four weeks, or six weeks) doable for you?
- Which activities and times worked best for you?
- Which did not work so well?
- Are you satisfied with your progress, your performance (how well you stuck with the program), and the results?

Once you've taken stock of the first 90 days of your walking-to-fitness journey, you can map out realistic goals and attainable activities for the next 90 days, working toward increasing your steps to 10,000 steps a day. Use the same strategies and tools you did for the first 12 weeks of the program—namely:

1. Decide whether you want to change your incremental goals (from or into one-week, two-week, three-week, four-week, or six-week segments).

2. Determine whether you want to change your daily steps goals—that is, the number of additional minutes of walking and additional steps per day—for Level Two. You should have recorded these goals on your Step Goals Worksheet before you started Level One.

3. Record any changes to your daily step goals on your Step Goals Worksheet.

4. Find new activities and strategies (such as a walking group) to keep you motivated.

5. Plan and schedule your daily walking exercise (or equivalent

Sample Step Goals Worksheet: Level Two

Level Two Goals
90-Day Goal: Add 2,000 exercise steps per day =11,000 total steps per day

Duration	Exercise Steps per day (baseline + exercise)	Steps per day	
Week 13	45 minutes	4,500	10,500
Week 14	45 minutes	4,500	10,500
Week 15	45 minutes	4,500	10,500
Week 16	45 minutes	4,500	10,500
Week 17	45 minutes	4,500	10,500
Week 18	45 minutes	4,500	10,500
Week 19	50 minutes	5,000	11,000
Week 20	50 minutes	5,000	11,000
Week 21	50 minutes	5,000	11,000
Week 22	50 minutes	5,000	11,000
Week 23	50 minutes	5,000	11,000
Week 24	50 minutes	5,000	11,000

Note: These figures are based on a moderate to brisk walking pace averaging about 100 steps a minute. For simplicity, the figures are rounded off; we suggest you do the same when setting your goals.

physical activities) on a week-by-week basis. Record these in the Activity Planner section of your Daily Step Log (or in your regular day planner). For best results, plan out your activities for the next week on the weekend of the current week.

6. Wear your Step-Counter every day, all day.

7. When you get the chance to sit it out or walk ... walk, adding

steps wherever you can to your daily life activities.

8. Record the number of steps taken each day in your Daily Step Log.

9. Continue to cut 100 excess calories a day, focusing on reducing simple sugars and fat in your diet.

Now, let's look at some ways to increase your daily steps—and, if you're ready, willing, and able, the intensity of your exercise as well.

Step-It-Up Strategies

You will no doubt enjoy some walking activities more than others. You might find some great for a while but boring as time goes by. Some will be simply more accessible to you than others. That's why it is important to add new walking activities that are doable and that interest you.

You should also keep in mind that not all steps are created equal. Depending on the terrain and the types of obstacles you come across in your daily travels, you may be burning far more calories than your Step-Counter leads you to believe. For instance, if your Step-Counter reads "1,710" steps for the day, you might conclude that you had an easy day. But if you took 192 of those steps from the street to the pedestal of the Statue of Liberty and another 192 steps back down to street level, that is a pretty good workout. (You'd have to be quite fit to make the whole 354-step ascent to the top of the statue, 22 stories from street level, but if you are moderately active and have no health problems, you could take the 192 stairs to the pedestal and then an elevator to the top.)

When it comes to burning calories, what you put into your steps can be just as important as how many steps you put in. Hills, stairs, snow, sand, and even grass place different and greater demands on your body, leading to more muscles being utilized and a greater amount of total calories burned.

Following are a few ways to increase the intensity of your walking. If you are significantly overweight or obese or have chronic health problems, check with your doctor before doing any activity in which you might increase your exertion levels.

The Need for Speed

For most people—particularly those who are sedentary or exercise lightly, have certain health problems, or are obese or significantly overweight—it is best to increase the duration, rather than the speed and intensity, of their exercise. But if you don't have a health reason why not to kick it up a notch, increasing both the speed and the duration of your walking will burn more calories much faster.

Walking briskly ($3\frac{1}{2}$ to 4 miles per hour) burns almost as many calories as jogging and can bring many of the same benefits. But even walking at a moderate pace or strolling brings benefits. A recent Harvard study of 40,000 female health professionals found that walking as little as an hour a week at any pace reduces the risk of heart disease, and that walking longer and faster produced an exponentially greater risk protection.

Here are a few tips for amping up your walking speed:

1. Take faster steps rather than longer strides. Lengthening your stride increases the strain on your legs and feet and can result in injury.

2. Use interval speeds. Walk slower for one interval and faster for another, and then rotate between the two intervals as you wish. For example, you can walk at a slower speed for 5 minutes, a faster speed for 5 minutes, and alternate speeds every five minutes. Or speed up for 1 or 2 minutes every 10 or 15 minutes. Or walk one slow mile and then one faster mile.

3. Pump your arms. Moving your arms vigorously will help accelerate your body forward and also works the upper body for additional cardiovascular benefits, and you'll burn 5 to 10% more calories to boot. Swing your arms naturally and in opposition to your legs, and pump from the shoulder (like race walkers do). Keep your elbow bent at about 90 degrees and close to your sides. Don't bend your wrists and clench your hands.

4. Use hand weights … cautiously. Using hand or wrist weights will increase your calorie usage, but they can alter your arm swing

and cause your wrists to bend, which can cause soreness or injury. If you feel strong enough to use them, start with one-pound weights and increase gradually, never using more than 10% of your body weight. Do not use hand weights if you have high blood pressure, heart disease, or other serious health problems.

Oh, Wizened Sand Walker

Loose, soft-packed sand is one of the most challenging surfaces to walk on, but the benefits are many. Walking on sand gives your heart, lungs, and legs a more intense workout than does walking on hard, smooth, level surfaces like asphalt, concrete, tile, and wood. Even though your pace will be slower, your heart rate will still climb as though you are doing a longer and more intense workout. In addition, the constant shifts in balance cause you to use core muscles throughout your trunk, making it a great workout for your abdominals as well. Plus, sand cushions the force of your foot as it strikes the ground, lessening the impact on your knees, ankles, and lower back.

When it comes to calorie-burning efficiency, walking on sand pays off in spades. According to a study published in the Journal of Science in Sports Medicine, walking on sand burns more than double the calories as walking on other surfaces. (No difference was found between running in sand with shoes or without them.)

Because sand-walking is more strenuous, yet gentle on your body, you can achieve a good, calorie-burning workout in less time and with less stress on your joints and feet. As an added benefit, you'll get to enjoy the fresh air and the views as you walk along the shore or around the lake.

Mount Rushmore = Mount Burn More

If you are one of those meanderers who plans your route to avoid hills and who makes a detour whenever one unexpectedly presents itself, you might want to consider this: Inclines pay major dividends.

>>**tip**

Use a retractable leash when walking the dog. It will help free your arms so that you can pump them more vigorously and burn more calories.

Walking hills is almost like a trip to the gym, but without the bad music, stretchy workout garb, and puddles of sweat. Walking on an incline causes a resistance in the muscles of your legs, and to a lesser extent in your stomach and buttocks, much the same way that lifting weights does. In fact, you will actually build muscle and gain strength with repeated hill climbs. Naturally, you also burn calories at a higher rate, and your lungs and heart get a better cardiovascular workout.

You don't have to walk up a steep incline or a hill measuring anything near the enormous height of Mount Rushmore (which, by the way, you couldn't actually walk up if you wanted to and would have to be a rock climber to scale if you could). Even gently rolling terrain can provide the muscle stimulus you need for extra calorie burning.

Incredibly, it is not just going up that provides this double-coupon of benefit. Walking downhill has its advantages as well. Doctors at the Voralberg Institute in Feldirch, Austria, examined two groups of people. One group walked up hills and took a tram to the bottom; the other took the tram up and walked down. The researchers were not expecting much from the downhill walking and were surprised to find that it significantly lowered blood sugar levels, a risk factor for Type II adult-onset diabetes. Uphill walking lowered triglycerides—fat in the blood, a risk factor for heart attacks—but did not have the same sugar-lowering effect as downhill walking. Both groups experienced lowered cholesterol levels, the uphill group more so than the downhill. Researchers concluded that the practice of downhill walking is a good starting point for people who are new to exercise.

However, walking downhill can put more stress on your knees and ankles than uphill walking does, which can cause muscle soreness and sometimes strains. So, make sure to keep your knees slight bent, to slow your pace, and to take shorter steps when descending an incline.

Calories Burned Walking

Walking Speed	Weight Calories Burned per mile						
	100 lbs.	120 lbs.	140 lbs.	160 lbs.	180 lbs.	200 lbs.	220 lbs.
2.0 mph	65	80	93	105	120	133	145
2.5 mph	62	74	88	100	112	124	138
3.0 mph	60	72	83	95	108	120	132
3.5 mph	59	71	83	93	107	119	130
4.0 mph	59	70	81	94	105	118	129
4.5 mph	69	82	97	110	122	138	151
5.0 mph	77	92	108	123	138	154	169

Walking uphill tends to be harder on your leg muscles. Of course, you want some extra tension (resistance) on those muscles. But to make it more comfortable and to prevent soreness or injury, lean forward slightly when walking uphill.

See? Hills really are your friends. Don't avoid them in your travels. Instead, charge after them—or, better yet, combine hills and flat terrains as a form of interval walking. You may hate them while you are climbing, especially at first, but you'll feel incredible when you hit the top. Remember, the more hills you take, the easier it will get. Meanwhile, you can take comfort in the good it's doing your body and pride in reaching higher.

>>tip

Save an old pair of walking shoes for your sandy strolls. Cushioning is not as crucial when walking on such a soft surface, and it will keep your regular shoes from getting wet with salt or lake water and for filling with painful grains of sand.

Stairs, Very Well and Good

You see them all the time and guiltily turn away—choosing, instead, to take the elevator or the escalator in favor of the stairway. Whether it's at the mall, your place of employment, the doctor's office, the library, the university, the municipal building, or wherever you have the choice to ride or walk, chances are, you ride.

Now, adding an extra 36 or so steps to your Step-Counter for the day might hardly seem worth walking up three stories for. But, as we've said, every step counts, and walking up stairs (and down, for that matter) counts almost double. Burning calories is what it's all about, and that's exactly what stairs do for you big time.

Climbing stairs is similar to lifting weights. In fact, a common leg exercise in the gym is called the "step-up" and is the exact motion of taking stairs; when you walk up stairs, the weight you are lifting is your own. A single step activates your quadriceps, hamstrings, calves, hip flexors, and dozens of smaller stabilizer muscles. Not only does this build muscle and expend calories, but it also improves bone density, which serves to stave off osteoporosis later in life.

Stair climbing is difficult, so add it to your daily regimen slowly and only if your health allows (check with your doctor if you have any concerns). For instance, if you work in a high-rise office building, walk a few floors and then catch the elevator. Increase the number of floors you walk every week.

Walking to Stand Still

Sometimes, the great outdoors is not so great for walking. In areas with hostile climates or for people who are incredibly busy, a home treadmill can be a convenient way to fit in a lot more steps. Besides convenience, treadmills tend to offer a bit more give and thus can be easier on your knees and ankles. On more advanced models, you can adjust the incline as well as keep track of your heart rate and the number of calories burned.

Treadmills have often been thought of as inferior to actually walking or running, but that has been proven false. One recent study showed no significant difference in the calorie-burning power of walking on a treadmill versus walking naturally. On top of that, a study conducted by researchers at the Medical College of Wisconsin in Milwaukee found that treadmills burned more calories than other home exercise machines, such as stationary bicycles, rowing machines, stair steppers, and cross-country ski machines.

Treading Water

Many athletes, such as runners and bicyclists, use "water jogging" (also called "aqua jogging") as one of their training exercises. You can add a toned-town version of this to your step activities, with much the same benefits.

Overuse injuries are rampant among runners, especially the obsessive types who refuse to let their bodies rest. Water jogging was created to give hurt runners an opportunity to maintain their fitness levels without exacerbating their injuries. Interestingly, the runners often found that after a session of water jogging they felt even stronger than they had before the injury that took them off the road.

> **" The elevator to success is out of order. You'll have to use the stairs ... one step at a time. "**
>
> *–Joe Girard*

You don't have to be an athlete to improve your fitness with water jogging (or walking). The natural resistance of the water cushions you from any impact and gives you a chance to strengthen myriad muscles (quadriceps, hamstrings, hip flexors, and core muscles). Plus, studies show you can burn up to 544 calories an hour while water jogging, which is nothing to scoff at.

You can water jog (or walk) a few different ways. One common method is to use a flotation belt or vest and walk or march in place in the deep end of the pool. Another method is to actually walk in a shallow lap lane with your feet on the floor and the water level

>>**tip**

anywhere from hip to chest high. The deeper you are, the more difficult it will be. You may want to use a pair of special pool shoes to protect your feet from abrasions.

When walking up and down hills, alternately pump your arms as though you were holding walking sticks or ski poles. (You can actually purchase trekking poles at specialty and some sporting goods stores.) This helps you get into a rhythm while you are ascending and burns more calories by activating muscles in your upper body.

No matter what form you use, concentrate on mimicking your usual land-walking style. Keep your head up and your eyes looking ahead. Push your feet directly down and back, and avoid using a circular, cycling-style leg motion. Take care not to fall into a lazy spasmodic form of treading water. Make sure to pump your arms while keeping a 90-degree bend in your elbows, and bring your knees all the way up to 90 degrees.

Walk Like an Alaskan

When you think of snowshoeing, you probably think of a lonely Grizzly Adams type, slowly trudging through the bleak landscape with things that resemble tennis rackets on his feet. You might be surprised to hear that the popularity of snowshoeing is on the rise. The development of high-tech, lightweight aluminum snowshoes and of competitive athletes discovering what an incredible form of cross-training snowshoeing is has brought this 6,000-year-old form of transportation back into vogue.

>>**tip**

If you find yourself using the rail for support or as an aid to help your ascension, try to switch off which arm you use, if possible (i.e., which side of the staircase you are on). This will help prevent any overuse injuries or asymmetrical muscle and strength development.

Snowshoeing combines many of the benefits of walking on sand and on hills. It combines a total-body, aerobic workout with serious strength and endurance training for your lower body and core muscles. If you add poles, it can also train the muscles of your back, shoulders, and arms. In fact, snowshoeing is such a great workout, it recently beat running in a head-to-head test of endurance and conditioning. A study published in the Journal of Sports Medicine and Physical Fitness pitted a group of runners against a group of snowshoers in a six-week contest to determine whose endurance and conditioning would improve the most. When the six weeks was over, both groups performed a test in which they ran and snowshoed to the point of exhaustion. The snowshoeing group lasted a whopping 44% longer than the runners before they were forced to stop.

Unlike cross-country skiing (another excellent variation of walking), snowshoeing does not have a learning curve. It requires little or no instruction and practice. Plus, in snowshoes, you can get to backcountry areas that cross-country skiers and snowmobilers cannot access.

Stair Mastering

Most gyms and community fitness centers have stair-stepping (also called stair-climbing and stair-treading) machines. Several manufacturers provide models you can purchase for home use, and you can also find them used—often barely used—on eBay and at garage sales. Just make sure any previously owned machines are in good repair before using. And it is always a good idea to try out a new piece of equipment at a gym or a friend's house before going to the expense of purchasing one.

Here are a few stair-stepping machine basics to remember:

- Begin with two 15-minute sessions a week, with a few days rest in between. Add five more minutes every week.

- Touch the handrails lightly for balance, but don't lean on them for support.

- Maintain good posture, with your head in alignment with your spine. Do not hunch over the machine.

- Start at a slow place and keep your foot on the pedal. Do not let your heels hang off the backs of the pedals.

- Take full steps, from 6 to 12 inches in height, depending on your strength and endurance. Do not make the itty-bitty baby steps you see in gyms so often.

- Don't forget to warm up before and to cool down after your walk or equivalent exercise activity.

Calories Burned in Alternate Activities

The following is a breakdown of the average calories burned per minute for people of varying weights for each activity listed.

Activity	130 lbs.	150 lbs.	180 lbs.
	Calories Burned per minute		
Aerobics (low impact)	4.9	5.9	7.2
Backpacking	6.9	8.2	10.1
Ballroom dancing (slow)	3.0	3.5	4.3
Basketball (casual)	6.9	8.2	10.1
Bicycling (light)	7.9	9.4	11.5
Cross-country skiing	13.2	17.1	18.8
Golf (hand cart)	4.4	4.7	5.6
Running (6-minute mile)	15.0	17.3	21.7
Stair-Climbing (moderate speed)	5.9	7.3	8.6
Swimming (fast)	9.8	11.3	13.5
Walking (flat surface, moderate pace)	4.7	5.4	6.5
Weight training	5.5	6.3	7.4

Many cross-country ski areas now have snowshoeing trails. If you live in or near an area that gets seasonal snow, you can snowshoe just about anywhere you know to be a safe place to walk or hike. (As a word of caution, just as you wouldn't want to walk or hike on a wet or icy path that is steep or slippery, you don't want to snowshoe in those areas either.)

Of course, not all of us have many opportunities to snow-shoe, just as we all can't get to the beach or to a lake easily. But if you ever have the chance to strap on a pair, don't miss the incredible exercise and the chance to explore some pristine snow-covered landscape.

The Sole of the Matter

Your body doesn't care if you walk barefoot in the sand or climb up the mountain in hiking boots,

Calories Burned Snowshoeing

You can burn 45% more calories snowshoeing than walking or running at the same speed. The following is the breakdown of calories burned per hour of snowshoeing for people of various weights:

Snowshoe Walking Level	120 lb.	150 lb.	180 lb.
	Calories Burned per hour		
Packed Flat	360	450	540
Packed hilly	410	515	620
Powder Rolling	560	700	840
Hilly with Poles	475	590	710

if you water jog in aqua socks or stroll through the mall in high-top sneakers. Wherever you walk, whatever way you walk, and however long you walk, walking and equivalent physical activity burns calories, strengthens muscles, and improves your cardiovascular health. And that bodes very well for you.

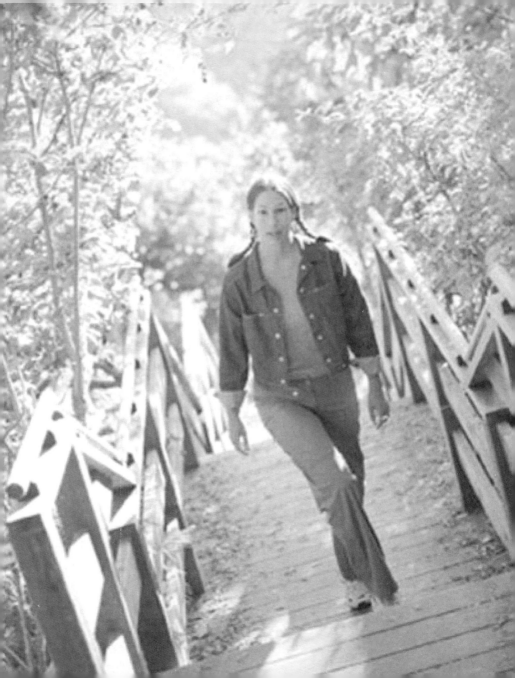

CHAPTER EIGHT

MIX IT UP

Variety: The Spice of Life … and Exercise

Keeping yourself motivated can be one of the most difficult challenges when trying to adopt any new habit. Exercise is no exception. Varying your walking routine, doing other types of exercise activities, and finding innovative ways to add steps to your regular life will help keep boredom at bay and you moving forward.

Everyone has their own likes and dislikes, and with the 10,000-Steps-A-Day Program you get to choose how you're going to get in your daily dose of physical activity. The good news is you've got plenty of choices. All you need to do is think about the different things that give you an emotional or physical lift, and then get creative in identifying ways to incorporate these "favorite things" into your physical activities.

Do you like sunrise, sunset, or the sun shining brightly in the heat of the day, or are you energized by moonlit nights? Are you drawn to streams, lakes, the ocean, the woods, the mountains, the desert? Do you fancy art, antiques, or architecture? Are you an amateur photographer, bird-watcher, or native plant enthusiast? Do you like to play tennis, golf, or volleyball?

Do you like to swim, skate, square dance? Do you like music or silence, socializing or solitude? All of these preferences and countless others provide myriad opportunities to personalize and to increase the pleasure quotient of your exercise activities.

If you start to feel like you're in an exercise rut, take some time to brainstorm specific new activities or variations in your current activities to spice it up. Jot down a list of new and different activities you'd like to add now or try later. Be creative, and don't limit yourself to "formal" types of exercise only; also come up with interesting ways to add steps to your daily life.

Every step you take is beneficial your health. Why not make at least some of them enjoyable too?

The Pleasure Principle

If it feels good, do it. Exercise is one of the few things in life in which you can follow that motto and not worry about what the neighbors or your mom will think. Not only that, but when exercise feels good, both physically and emotionally, you will do it, again and again, and not to give up on it.

Here are a few ways to perk up your walking:

Alter your walking route. Go the opposite direction, starting where you usually end. Turn left where you would normally turn right. Go a block farther.

Use the buddy system. Find a walking partner, join a walking club, or form a new group with friends, neighbors, or coworkers. Create a competition to see who can add the most steps in three months (or more or less), and chip in with your partners to fund a small prize. Ask someone who is in a slump to join you and be their walking mentor, or choose a partner who is near or a bit beyond your level to inspire you.

Take a walking tour of your city. Many cities have tours of historic districts, theater districts, manufacturing districts (for example, fashion and glass-making), and other special-interest areas. Most also have walking tours of local gardens and "dream" homes. Or just take a sidewalk tour of a neighborhood of interesting or quaint homes. Don't restrict yourself only to your neighborhood; go where the walking and gazing are good. As long as you park in a public place, don't trespass, and don't act like you're casing the joint, no one will care if you walk and look.

Tour a vineyard. Winery hopping seems to have become one of America's favorite pastimes. If you are so inclined, add a walk through the vineyard to your next stop at the local winery or when you visit wineries in other places.

Tour a farm or factory. Many factories and some larger farms have regularly scheduled tours. Many others give tours on a call-ahead basis. Arrange and chaperone the tour for your child's class (with the school's

FitnessFACT

Thinking on Your Feet

Walking is very good for the brain. By increasing breathing and heart rate, walking increases blood circulation and the amount of oxygen and glucose to the brain. This enhances the use of energy to fuel the body and also improves the body's ability to remove waste. Walking doesn't suck up the extra oxygen and glucose that other forms of more strenuous exercise do. While you walk, you are effectively "oxygenating" your brain—which gives proof to the old saying that walking "clears your head." So, when you're faced with a stressful or complex situation that requires your concentration and some brain power, take a walk. Chances are, the answers will come to you, and you will no doubt feel calmer and more confident about it too.

cooperation, of course). Tour a farm at harvest time, and go through the corn maze for extra steps.

Take a walking vacation. A whole segment of the travel industry is devoted to arranging walking tours around the globe. London. Paris. Tuscany. Toronto. Boston. New York. Maui. Just pick your destination and call your travel agent or a walking tour guide.

Go on an art walk. Even small towns host tours of artists' homes, studios, and galleries, and you can often walk at least parts of the tour.

Go to the farmer's market, craft show, or county fair. While getting in a good walk in a lively environment, you can also check out and purchase the works of local craftspeople and pick up some fresh and organic food products too.

Go to a home and garden show or a boat show. Do a complete lap around the facility before stopping at any exhibits.

Go window shopping in a new place. Head to the big city, or a large mall, or an outdoor shopping center, or a factory outlet complex—somewhere you don't usually frequent that has lots of interesting stores and a safe, pleasant environment.

Visit the zoo or aquarium. This is a great way to get exercise with (or without) the kids.

Visit museums and art galleries. Yes, it is possible to walk and look at the same time. When you see a work of art that captivates you, you can circle the room to see it from different angles or pace in front of it.

Go antiquing. Many towns have antique districts, where you will find shop after shop within walking distance.

Stroll through an arboretum, botanical garden, or nature preserve. Soak in nature and breathe free air as you walk.

Walk through a college or university campus. Many are accessible to the public during the day, have well-maintained walking paths and sidewalks, and are filled with interesting architecture and gorgeous landscaping.

Walk around the track. Go to a nearby public school—when classes are out, of course—and do walking laps around the track. Four laps equals about 2,000 steps.

Participate in a charity walk. This gives new meaning to the saying, "Do well by doing good," benefiting your health while benefiting your community.

*"Perhaps the truth depends on
a walk around the lake."*

—*Wallace Stevens*

Hike a wilderness trail. Virtually every region in the United States has hiking trails, and you can usually find guidebooks with maps to popular and accessible sites at your local library, bookstores, and specialty walking/hiking stores. Many state and municipal tourism boards and chambers of commerce also provide such materials. Go in the spring to view blossoming trees and wild flowers. In autumn, enjoy colored leaves and gather pinecones. In summer, hike along a creek or river, or to a lake or waterfall. In the winter, strap on some snowshoes and traverse the winter wonderland.

Volunteer to walk dogs. Animal shelters are always looking for help caring for unwanted and stray pets. Friends, family, and neighbors often appreciate a hand with this too.

Volunteer to walk shut-ins. Check with local nursing and assisted-care facilities to see whether you can push people in wheelchairs around the facility, indoors or outside.

Form a litter patrol. Organize your family or a group of neighbors into teams to walk around the neighborhood or community playgrounds, parks, and sporting fields and pick up debris.

Take your family on a holiday walk of lights. December is a good time for evening strolls around the neighborhood to check out the holiday light displays. The kids will get a better view than when

Activity Step Conversions

Activity	Steps per minute		Activity	Steps per minute	
	Female	Male		Female	Male
Aerobic Dance (low impact)	142	127	Lawn Darts	71	73
Backpacking (hilly, < 10 lb. load)	189	181	Pilates	94	91
			Racquetball (casual)	189	181
Badminton	71	73	Skating, ice (casual)	189	181
Baseball	142	127	Skating, inline	200	190
Basketball (casual)	165	127	Skiing (casual but not bunny slope)	165	145
Bicycling (light)	142	145			
Bicycling, stationary	189	181	Snowshoeing	212	199
Bocce Ball	71	73	Soccer (casual)	189	181
Bowling	71	73	Stair Machine	236	218
Canoeing	94	91	Stairs, down	71	73
Dancing, (fast)	118	109	Stairs, up	212	199
Dancing, (slow)	71	73	Swimming (freestyle)	189	181
Football (flag/touch)	212	199	Tennis (singles)	212	199
Gardening (moderate)	118	109	Volleyball	118	91
			Waterskiing	165	145
Horseshoes	71	73	Weight lifting	71	73
Judo / Karate	260	264	Yoga	71	54
Jumping Rope (slow)	212	199			

> **It's All Relative**
>
> 2,000 steps = Walking through the mall for 20 minutes without pausing
> 2,000 steps = Walking 1 mile
> 10,000 steps = Walking 5 miles

riding in a car, and you'll get to see their reactions.

Turn your walk into a family game. Bring the kids and play "I Spy" as you walk. Or make it into a scavenger hunt, which will take just a little planning ahead (a list and fanny packs or back packs for carting around treasures).

Of course, we realize that you can't take one of these special walking excursions every day of the week. But if you make an effort to schedule one such "fun walk" once a week, or every other week, or once a month, it will give you something to look forward to, help keep you motivated, and increase your enjoyment in walking. Think of these outings as

Step Insteads

Sure, walking is an all-around great form of exercise. It is an effective way to lose weight and improve your health. It is easy and inexpensive to do. And it is genuinely enjoyable to many people. But what if you're just not that into it? No problem. You can substitute some of your walking activities with other forms of exercise that you are into.

Golf, for example, one of America's favorite pastimes, is a great way to crank up the steps—provided you use your feet and not a motorized cart to get around the course. Regulations state that a 9-

>>tip

Pedal Counts

Bicycling is a good way to vary your routine and it is an acceptable substitute for walking when soreness or an injury makes walking uncomfortable or impossible. Just attach your Step-Counter to your shoe and pedal away. But be aware that you will log fewer steps on your Step-Counter than had you walked the same distance or for the same period of time. To get the maximum calorie-burning and fitness benefits from your bike ride, pedal all or most of the time; don't just coast for stretches, unless you're very tired.

hole course must be at least 2,600 yards in length, the equivalent of 3,900 steps. A regulation 18-hole course must be 5,200 yards long, which equates to about 7,800 steps. Even the small pitch-n-putt courses are good for about 1,500 steps. Add to that the calories consumed lugging a bag or pushing it in a hand cart, swinging the club, and cursing and hopping up and down when you miss the put, and you are in for a mammoth calorie burn.

If your thing isn't golf—which, for all its popularity, does have its own downsides (a bunch of expensive equipment, pricey greens fees, competing for tee times, the frustration of honing a difficult skill, the length of time it takes to play a round of golf)—there are plenty of other fitness activities that you can do in place of or in addition to some of your walking sessions.

A few common examples of "instead" physical activities and their corresponding steps-per-minute equivalency follow. Please

> **" *There are many ways of going forward, but only one way of standing still.* "**
>
> –*Franklin D. Roosevelt*

note that this is an average. Generally speaking, the conversion will be slightly higher for women and slightly lower for men. Weight, body composition, age, physical condition, and other factors can also affect the step-count equivalency.

Life Steps

Opportunities to add steps are everywhere you are during the course of your day—as you take care of your family, do your household chores, run errands, commute, work, socialize with friends, go to church or school, and help others in your community. Pay attention as you go about your daily life and notice those times that you are idle when you could be stepping or at least standing. Look for opportunities where you can walk rather than ride or sit and where you can take more steps rather than short cuts.

For example, rather than stopping at the drive-through Java Hut on your way to work, take a 10-minute walk and bring a cuppa home-brewed Joe with you. Walk around the house or your yard while you talk on the phone. Pace or stand during meetings. Step in place as you watch TV. Idle steps are everywhere, just waiting for you to discover and claim them, and it all adds up. The more steps you take, the more calories you burn, taking you closer to your optimal weight and better health.

Remember to wear your Step-Counter all day every day and to record your total daily steps, ensuring that you're getting an accurate count of, and giving yourself credit for, all of the steps you're taking to improve your fitness. Also, make sure to take notice of the intensity of your physical activities, stepping it up a notch whenever you can and giving yourself credit for that extra effort too. You might find it useful to record this information in your Daily Step Log.

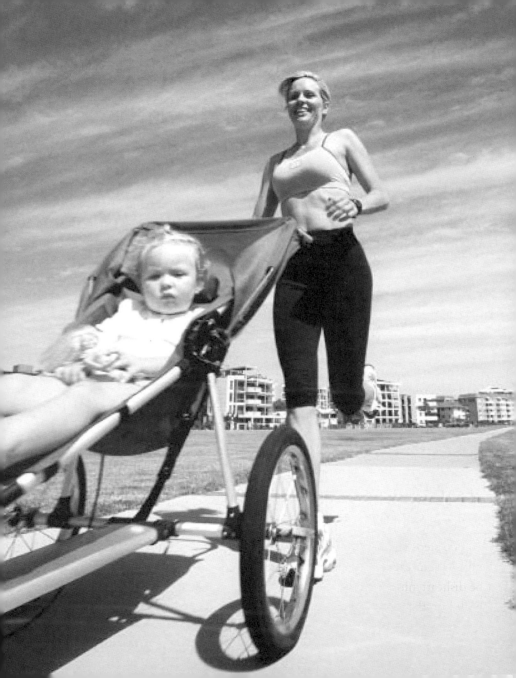

CHAPTER NINE

STAY ON TRACK

Rebound, Recovery, and Contingency Plans

Life happens. And sometimes it gets in the way of your exercise. On "down" days, busy days, sick days, travel days, and holidays, getting in a brisk 30-minute walk or even a 5-minute stroll can be a challenge. Inevitably, a time will come when it just doesn't happen, when something else in your life takes priority. That is to be expected, and it's okay. After all, the best exercise program is one that fits into your life, not one that you fit your life around.

What you don't want, though, is to take too long of a break or too many breaks too often. Repeatedly stopping and starting an exercise program is a lot like playing the lottery, with equally disappointing and frustrating results. Your chances of hitting the jackpot—or, in this case, your goal of 10,000 steps and a trimmer, healthier body—are slim to none. Prolonged lulls in your exercise routine will interfere with your progress, and no doubt be disheartening, making it even more difficult to get over the slump and back into the groove of exercising.

" Obstacles are those frightful things you see when you take your eyes off your goal. "

—Henry Ford.

If you skip a day, try not to skip two. If an important obligation or health issue unavoidably takes you away from your normal exercise routine for longer than that, try to find an interim physical activity that you are able to do. If getting away for even 10 minutes of exercise is not possible, at least try to increase your steps as you go about your life. Better yet, try to do both.

The key to keeping the momentum going with your 10,000-Steps-A-Day Program is to prepare for those times when life throws a wrench in your exercise routine—as it assuredly will at some point, just as it does for everyone, including top athletes and super models. Perhaps the most important advance preparation you can do is psychological—getting rid of the all-or-nothing mindset that so often derails people when they hit a road block or a rough patch. Your goal should be to get back with the program as soon as possible, which might mean doing less exercise or reducing the intensity of your exercise for a while. Even during the worst of times, you can usually fit in 5 or 10 minutes of some form of physical activity. Since walking is one of the most flexible and least strenuous forms of exercise, you should be able to get in your steps somehow.

Also watch out for "never" and "can't" thinking—the Achilles heel of those new or returning to exercise, who tend to panic if they lose a little ground before the activity has had a chance to set. If you keep telling yourself that you'll "never get back to exercising regularly," or that "it's too hard to get back in the groove," or that you "just can't do it," you'll start believing it … and then your actions (in this case, inaction) will follow suit. That kind of self-defeating thinking is like shooting yourself in the foot.

So, try to think positive … and to think ahead. Don't let a set-back sabotage your exercise program. Do some brainstorming upfront or as soon as an obstacle arises to come up with creative ways to keep you moving or to get you moving again when life sidetracks or sidelines you with illness, injury, or other priorities. Missing a day or two of walking once in a while is no big deal. Neither is slowing down on your exercise for a while. In fact, it will happen. You can plan on it. And you'd be wise to plan for it.

Name that Saboteur

Chances are this is not the first exercise program you've undertaken. Like most people, you've probably started and stopped a few different ones, trying to find one that would stick. You might even have another exercise activity that works well for you right now and are simply looking to expand your fitness horizons with the 10,000-Steps-A-Day Program. Regardless, through your past experience you probably know which obstacles are most likely to disrupt your exercise routine. For most people, the barriers that usually cause them to skip or stop exercising are the ones they put up themselves and can take down themselves, provided they are motivated enough to do it. Some obstacles, though, are unpreventable. That does not mean they are immovable.

Take a few minutes to identify the obstacles that are most likely to trip you up, and then be proactive in thinking up ways to remove them. Here are some common exercise barriers and maneuvers for getting over and around them.

1. My walking partner cancelled. Ask a coworker, friend, neighbor, or your spouse to fill in. Take a different route at a different time, if need be. If you can't find someone to walk with you, do one of your "fall-back" physical activities that you can do alone instead.

2. I'm too tired. Because exercise increases the production of endorphins, it can actually give you an energy boost when you're tired. If you're dog tired or genuinely fatigued, try walking a shorter distance and on a smooth flat surface, or try a different low-key activity, like bowling or walking in place while you watch your favorite 30-minute TV program or during the commercials of a 60-minute program. Go to bed earlier, and try getting up 10 to 30 minutes earlier and getting in your walking then.

3. I'm not feeling well. Some illnesses do require bed rest, and your first priority must be to give your body what it needs to heal. In

FitnessFACT
Walking for Two

Pregnant women do not get enough exercise—in part due to the misconception that pregnancy is a physical disability that limits or inhibits physical activity. In reality, most expectant mothers would benefit from doing moderate exercise regularly throughout most of their pregnancies. According to a study by the St. Louis University School of Public Health, only 1 in 6 pregnant women get sufficient exercise, and only 16% get the recommended 30 minutes of exercise at least 5 days a week, as compared with 27% of non-pregnant women. Moderate to brisk walking has been cited by numerous studies as a safe and comfortable way for expectant moms to get in their daily exercise.

many cases, though, you can adapt the duration and intensity of your walking to suit your physical condition. And you can usually add at least some steps by walking around the house.

4. I'm working extra hours. Far too often, far too many of us are going in early, staying late, working through lunch, and not taking breaks during the workday. Try to make this exception rather than the rule of your work life. Always take your full lunch break and use 10 minutes of it to get away from your desk and to walk around the building, whether inside or out. When possible, stand rather than sit, pace rather than stand, and walk to a coworker's desk rather than emailing, phoning, or using the intercom.

5. I can't find childcare. Take the little ones on a walk with you, or to the park or playground, or just outside in the backyard or to the basement or play room. And actually play with them. Many childhood games—such as tag, ring-around-the-rosy, red rover, hop

scotch, and simply tossing a beach ball or batting a balloon back and forth—provide low-impact aerobic exercise, and will give you some fun one-on-one time with your kids.

6. I have an injury that makes walking difficult or painful. Switch your focus from what you can't do to what you can do, and adapt your physical activity accordingly. It doesn't have to be a brisk 30-minute walk; it can be water jogging or swimming a few laps around the pool, or a 10-minute ride on a stationery bike, or whatever physical activity doesn't hurt you or aggravate your injury. Contrary to popular belief, exercise should not be painful.

7. I have house guests. Ask them to join you on your regular walk. Or set your alarm so that you can rise before your guests do and get in your walk then. Or plan an excursion that involves walking, such as visit to a nearby museum, botanical garden, or unique shopping district.

8. I'm busy with a holiday or special event. If you're busy shopping, running errands, doing extra household chores, you're probably adding lifestyle steps that will help compensate for some of the time it takes away from your regular walking routine. Try to add as many extra steps into these chores and preparations as you can, for example, by parking at the far end of the lot or walking the dog an extra 10 minutes. Also try to incorporate a physical activity into your holiday activities, such as a walk around the block to check

out the Christmas lights or a trip to the zoo for a child's birthday.
9. My family (kids and/or spouse) needs more time with me. The
solution to this is kind of a no-brainer, isn't it? Simply go for a
walk together. Yet, many people fail to do that—either because
they treasure their daily walk as "their" time, or their loved one(s)
aren't interested in walking ("It's b-o-r-i-n-g," is a common
response), or they just didn't think about it. Find an activity that
involves walking, or any physical activity, that you all do enjoy, and
schedule one or two such activities every week. Shoot hoops, hula
hoop, go bike riding, or do yard work together.
10. An important personal or professional obligation conflicts with
my walking routine. The great thing about walking is that you don't
have to do it at a specific time or place, or for a specific block of time
or for a specific duration or intensity. You can improvise. You can
reschedule. You can break it up into smaller pieces. You can add more
steps to your regular life, for example, by walking to the school for a
parent-teacher conference, around the field as you watch your child
play soccer, or to lunch with your coworkers. You can walk around
the building before or after that important meeting, or walk on the
treadmill at home or in the hotel when your workday finally ends.
11. I'm traveling on business. Make it a point to always pack your
walking shoes, sports socks, fanny pack, whistle and/or cell phone,
and Step-Counter. Choose a hotel with a gym or at least a pool,

and fit some exercise in around your work schedule. Rather than ordering in, eating in the hotel's restaurant, or driving with clients to lunch or dinner, walk to a nearby restaurant. If possible, arrive a few hours earlier or stay a few hours later than necessary, and take a walking tour of the area.

12. I'm going on vacation with family or friends. Vacations provide countless opportunities for new and enjoyable walking excursions and physical activities; just plan ahead and include activities that get you up off your duff and moving in your itinerary. The best way to really experience a place is to walk it, so make sure to plan walking tours of interesting areas and sites. There are travel organizations that host safe and fascinating guided walking tours of hot travel destinations around the globe.

13. The weather outside is frightful. Whether it's too hot, too cold, too wet, too windy, or too slippery for your tastes, you've got two choices: wear clothing that is appropriate for the weather or head inside to exercise. Or, you can do a combination of the two.

>> **tip**

Have Shoes, Will Walk

Unexpected opportunities to walk for 10 or 15 minutes pop up all the time. Be prepared to get your steps when the getting is good. Keep an older pair of sneakers (with a clean pair of sports socks stuck inside) in your backpack, carry-on luggage, or your car.

Sure Cures for the Summertime Blues

Heat has a way of sneaking up and packing a wallop before you even realize it's having an effect on you. Though you might notice that you're sweating a lot or feeling flushed, you'll probably be unaware of the toll that excessive heat is taking on your body until you've already overdone it. Overexerting in hot or humid conditions can overtax your internal temperature-regulation system, which puts extra stress on your cardiovascular system.

To dissipate heat, the heart circulates more blood through the skin, which consequently makes less blood available to muscles. So, your heart rate will be higher when you walk on a hot day (or on a treadmill in an overheated room) than it would in a cooler environment. If the humidity is also high, it will put added stress on your body, because sweat doesn't evaporate as quickly from your skin under humid conditions. Then, your body temperature rises in response to both the exercise and to the higher air temperature. This can lead to dehydration, muscle cramps, heat exhaustion, and heat stroke.

Here are some suggestions for avoiding these heat-related conditions:

1. Drink enough water. Your body can lose up to 2 quarts of fluid per hour when exerting in heat. In addition to water, sports drinks and diluted fruit juices are fine, but stay away from sugared and

caffeinated drinks. If you walk briskly for 30 or more minutes in the heat, you might want to consider a sports drink, which contains electrolytes (chloride, potassium, and sodium) that you lose through sweating.

2. Walk in the morning or early evening, when the temps are cooler.

3. Walk in the shade, when you can.

4. Walk inside an air-conditioned building. A brisk walk through the mall or a moderately paced walk through an art gallery or museum are good substitutes for balmy days.

5. Wear breathable, lightweight, light-colored, loose-fitting clothing. Loose, breathable clothing allows more air to pass over your skin, aiding in sweat evaporation and cooling your body. Avoid clothing made with heavy, dark, nonporous, and rubberized material, which can impede sweat evaporation and increase your body temperature.

6. Wear a baseball cap or sun hat and sunglasses, to limit your exposure to the blaring sun and damaging UV rays.

7. Decrease your exertion level. Walk for a shorter distance or period of time and at a slower pace. If you normally do interval walking—for example, walking at a slower pace for the first 5 minutes, then faster for 20 minutes, then slower for the last 5 minutes—try walking at a moderate pace for the whole 30 minutes. Or set a distance, rather than a timed goal, for example, walk 1 mile or around the block.

8. Give your body time to adapt to higher temperature. If you are generally healthy and reasonably fit, your body will usually get used to the heat so that you can exercise without your body temperature and heart rate rising excessively. For the first week or two of hot weather, shorten the length of your walk and walk slower, and then gradually increase your distance and exertion.

9. Substitute an activity that won't heat you up. Take a swim in a cool lake or swim in a pool in the evening or inside an air-conditioned building. Plan a weekend hike in the woods and mountains, where the shade and higher elevation will be cooler (but don't hike at too high of an elevation in the heat, which can be hard on your body too).

10. Check with your doctor if you have a chronic health problem or take medications. Heat can cause adverse reactions in combination with certain medications, such as antihistamines and diuretics.

Winter Wise

When a chill nips the air and the daylight hours shrink considerably, it can be tempting to swap your morning or evening walk for a hot cup of tea in a recliner by the fire. Don't let a little thing like winter weather make you a shut-in. With the right clothing, some ingenuity, and a few safety precautions, you can have your walk and your hot toddy too. By staying on track with your 10,000 Steps-A-Day Program throughout the cool season, you'll be a step ahead when warm weather breaks and it's time to bring out the warm-weather "skinny" clothes. Plus, being physically active will help keep your energy and strength up while helping to stave off the cold-weather blues and those extra pounds so many people gain during the winter.

The winter months are a great time to start adding calisthenics and strength training to improve your flexibility, strength, and stamina. You might also want to take the opportunity to try some outdoor snow activities, like snowshoeing and cross-country skiing, as well as new indoor activities, such as swimming, yoga, using a treadmill or stair stepper, and mall walking.

That said, with today's weather-resistant apparel, you can comfortably and safely walk outside on cold, wet, or windy days. Here are some guidelines that will help keep you warm, dry, and protected:

• Check the weather report. Decrease the odds of getting caught outside in a blizzard, a downpour of freezing rain, excessive wind, or below-freezing temperatures.

• Don't forget to take any wind chill into consideration. If the temperature dips far below zero or is below minus 20 degrees with a wind chill, choose an inside activity instead, or skip a day and

FitnessFACT
Separating Fat from Myth

When you stop exercising, your muscles turn to fat. True or false?

First, exercise isn't something you start and stop, or shouldn't be. It should be a healthy habit you adopt for life. That said, if you do stop exercising, you will lose muscle and the rate at which you burn calories will also drop, which can indeed make you gain fat. But muscle doesn't turn into fat. It is simply not possible; they are two totally different types of body tissue. And nobody turns to flabby blubber overnight; overeating and not exercising over time does that. Nor does getting rotund and mushy mean you're doomed to stay that way. Even the Pillsbury Doughboy could slim down and tone up by cutting calories and exercising regularly.

get in as many extra steps around your work and home as you can.

- Dress in layers. Start with a thin first layer of long underwear made of synthetic micro-fibers, such as polypropylene, which wick sweat away from your body. The second layer is for insulation; try light-weight fleece or wool, preferably with a zipper that you can open to release excess body heat and per-spiration. The third layer should be wind- and water-proof, or at least resistant. An outer layer made of GoreTex® (or a similar material) and a down liner is ideal, providing excellent protection without excess weight. If you get too warm, you can open or shed the third or second layer.

- Wear appropriate footwear. You'll need a good-fitting pair of walking shoes or hiking boots with a water resistant upper sole and good traction on the bottom to prevent slipping. Use wool socks or socks made with a blend of cotton and propylene fibers.

Signs of Heat Exhaustion and Heat Stroke

Immediately stop walking if you experience the following symptoms while exercising in hot weather. Get out of the heat, drink water, elevate your feet above your head, place wet cloths on your skin (particularly the back of your neck), and seek medical help.

Heat Exhaustion		Heat Stroke	
Cool, clammy skin	Weakness	Hot, flushed, dry skin	Nausea
Muscle cramps	Disorientation	Little or no	Feeling Faint
Weak pulse	Headache	perspiration	Dizziness
Nausea	Shortness of	Very high body	Weakness
Chills	Breath	temperature	Confusion/delirium
Dizziness		(104 to 106 F)	Headache
		Shortness of Breath	

If you wear 2 layers of socks, wear the thinner layer closest to your skin; silk and silk-blend socks make a good inner layer of sock. Also make sure that your shoes are not too tight, which can impede circulation, making your feet even colder.

• Wear gloves. Like your feet, your hands are not well insulated parts of your body and are usually more sensitive to cold and more prone to the ill effects of winter weather, such as frostbite. Wearing a polypropylene glove liner will give you extra protection. In extreme cold and in very wet or snowy conditions, layer your gloves like you do the rest of your body, with the thin sweat-wicking layer first, then a warm insulating layer like wool, with a wind- and water-resistant layer (such as a ski glove) on top.

• Cover your head and neck. Much of your body heat will escape

FitnessFACT

The word "exercise" derives from the Latin root meaning "to maintain, to keep, to ward off." Walking regularly, through every season, will help you to maintain your weight, to keep you on track with your fitness goals, and to ward off health problems.

through head unless you wear a warm hat; wool or fleece is best. A neck scarf will also help you to retain body heat and to stay comfortable. In wet weather, you can layer a beanie under a hood or a hat made out of a water-resistant material. Hats with masks that cover the face are also recommended for windy and very cold weather.

- Protect yourself from the sun. It may not look like it on many winter days, but the sun is there and its rays can still do damage to skin and eyes. Wear sunscreen, especially at high altitudes, and lip balm with sunscreen, especially when it is windy, and sunglasses or goggles.
- Warm up. Walk in place for a few minutes and do a few gentle stretches before you start to walk or snowshoe or whatever winter activity suits your fancy. Start out at a slow pace and gradually increase your speed.
- Make sure you're visible. With shorter, more foggy, and more overcast days, you could well find yourself walking in the dark or in reduced visibility conditions.
- Walk when it's light and the visibility is good when possible, and always wear reflective clothing so drivers can see you.
- Start out facing the wind, while you have the most energy and

> **"He who limps is still walking. "**
>
> *—Stanislaw J. Lee*

body heat. That way, the wind will be at your back for the last half of your walk, when you're the most likely to be sweaty and consequently more vulnerable to frostbite.

• Pay attention to where you're walking. Watch out for wet and slippery surfaces, including "black ice," deep snow, and thin ice that might break, submersing your feet (or worse, your body) in freezing water.

• Give your body sufficient fuel. Dehydration increases your risk of frostbite, so make sure to drink enough water, and avoid ca feinated and alcoholic beverages, which accelerate dehydration. Eat nutritiously to make sure your body has enough energy to function efficiently. A small snack comprised of protein and complex carbs 30 to 45 minutes before walking is also a good idea.

• Watch your breathing. If you smoke or have asthma or a lung condition such as chronic pleurisy, pay close attention to your breathing when walking in the cold. Both exercise and cold can induce asthma attacks, so it is wise to wear a face mask or scarf over your mouth so that the air entering your lungs is warmer and to always carry your asthma medication.

• Take shorter walks. Limit your exposure to extreme cold to 10 to

Signs of Frostbite and Hypothermia

Following the guidelines, above, will keep you healthy and safe while keeping you on track with your 10,000-Steps-A-Day Program. But these warning signs of the potential ill effects of prolonged exposure to severe cold are always good to know.

Frostbite: Begins as patch of white or pale skin, accompanied by loss of feeling or sharp stinging, usually on face, fingers, and/or toes. After mild frostbite, when the body warms and blood returns to the frozen area, the white patch becomes red and swollen, and it burns or stings. With a severe case, the skin might turn purple or black and will be extremely painful when rewarmed, and requires medical attention.

Hypothermia: Usually begins with intense shivering, loss of coordination, and inability to do complex tasks and progresses to slurred speech, mental confusion, and memory loss. This is a serious medical emergency that requires immediate attention.

30 minutes at a time, depending on the weather conditions. Your extremities are particularly vulnerable to losing their heat, which is uncomfortable, and to frostbite, which is painful and destroys tissue.

• Wear a helmet for winter sports, such as tobogganing, ice skating, snowshoeing, snowboarding, and skiing. Ice can do some real damage if you take a spill, and snow is much harder when your

>>tip

Just Say No to Fatigue

If you feel too fatigued to walk, or start off on your walk only to realize after a few minutes that you're too fatigued to continue, listen to your body. Slow down. Turn around and cut it short. Or skip day and try again tomorrow. If you consistently feel worn out during or after your walking exercise, cut back 20 to 50%, both in duration and intensity, for a while, until you're feeling better. Then, once you're in the pink again and your energy starts returning, gradually build back up to your pre-fatigue levels. Remember, don't give up … just tone it down.

head smacks it than you might think.

- Walk or exercise indoors. Any aerobic activity you can do for 30 minutes at a time or for shorter intervals that combine to make 30 minutes of exercise a day.
- Sign up for a Pilates or fencing class at the community college. Join an adult basketball league through your local community center or church. Buy a treadmill or stationery bike, and get in your steps while you watch TV in the evening. Take a swim at the local Y, or join a health club. Whatever works for you…just keep moving and keep moving forward toward your optimal weight and 10,000 steps a day.

CHAPTER TEN

WARNING: EXCESS FAT IS HARMFUL TO YOUR HEALTH

The Dangerous Link between Obesity and Chronic Illness ... and How You Can Break It

Our nation—and to a slightly lesser extent, much of the industrialized world—is facing a serious health crisis. You can see it everywhere, in the malls, churches, factories, office buildings, and, unfortunately, in the schoolyards and playgrounds of each and every state. This crisis is obesity, and it is associated with a host of serious, debilitating and life-threatening health problems.

About 3 in 10 Americans are obese—31% of the population, some 59 million people, among them children and adolescents. In fact, the rate of obesity among children and adolescents has nearly doubled in the past 20 years, to 13%.

Obesity is generally defined as being at least 30 pounds overweight; it is also commonly defined as being more than 20% for men and 25% for women above the maximum desired weight for a specific height. The more overweight the person is, the higher her or his risk of serious chronic conditions, such as type-2 diabetes, heart disease, high blood pressure, and osteoarthritis.

Obesity is also associated with a higher morbidity rate. For example, men who are severely obese have a life expectancy of 13 years less than men of normal weight, reports the Journal of the American Medical Association. Anyone who is 60 or more pounds overweight is considered "severely obese," 100 pounds or more overweight is considered "morbidly obese," and 200 pounds or more is considered "super obese."

Obesity is associated with more than 300,000 American deaths each year, according to the U.S. Centers for Disease Control. Lack of regular physical activity is responsible for 250,000 deaths a year. Not surprisingly, obesity and inactivity usually go hand-in-hand.

There has been much discussion and many studies trying to pinpoint which comes first, obesity or inactivity. The two are so closely linked that it's like trying to resolve the old chicken-and-egg debate. One thing is clear: the more inactive you are, the more weight you gain; the more weight you gain, the more sedentary you become.

Lack of exercise, though a primary factor in obesity, is not the sole cause. Overeating and poor nutrition are also major contributors. Age, genetics, and basic human biology each play a role as well. Some medications (such as corticosteroids) and underlying medical conditions (such as hormonal disorders) can also contribute to a person's tendency to become obese.

There are many things we can do to improve our eating and exercise habits. Taking those measures seriously and making them a part of our everyday habits for life will help to offset the natural effects of aging and to reduce the risk of chronic illness. We're stuck with our basic biology, though, and the best we can do is try to understand it and work with what evolution has given us.

Here's the deal, and frankly, it's kind of a raw one: We all still harbor our Paleolithic DNA—the internal "program" that drives the physiological functions that helped early humans survive famine, predators, and hostile environments. Our prehistoric ancestors spent all day every day foraging for food. Their daily activity was extremely vigorous and their food intake was minimal. When they went without sustenance, their bodies would slow down their metabolisms to burn fewer calories in an effort to sustain them until they could eat again. When they did come upon food, they would gorge themselves, somehow knowing that many of the calories would be stored as fat—a valuable commodity and energy source when you get only one small meal every few days. Similarly, early humans cultivated a taste for sweet things, because bitter flavors often turned out to be poisonous.

Fast forward almost 4 million years to the early and mid-1900s. Though food was a lot more plentiful and meals more regular then, people were still getting plenty of exercise through farming and manual labor. Human diets still consisted of primarily whole foods—fresh meat, poultry, fish, vegetables, grains, fruits, nuts, and seeds—with very few preserved foods, small amounts of sugar and salt, and virtually no processed foods. Though these forebears looked quite different from their cave-dwelling ancestors, on a cellular level, they were almost identical.

> **"Walking is man's best medicine."**
>
> *–Hippocrates*

Now, move the clock forward just 100 or so years to the present day, and we are in the midst of a full-blown catastrophe. We still have the primal urge to gorge ourselves when we get hungry, yet in our daily lives we do a fraction of the physical activity that our DNA is programmed for and our bodies are designed for. We no longer have to walk long distances and do physical labor to get our food. Only a small percentage of us have physically demanding jobs; in fact, the majority of us sit on our duffs all day every day while we earn a buck. Meanwhile, food is plentiful, but lacking in nutrition and loaded with fat and sugar.

The basic nutritional needs of most people are approximately

2,000 calories a day for women and 2,500 for men. More active people, those who exercise vigorously on a regular basis and manual laborers, for example, may need 4,000 or more calories a day. Pregnant women and nursing mothers need about 300 to 500 more calories a day than other women. Because the body cannot store carbohydrates or proteins, it converts anything we don't immediately use to fat, which is stored in the body as an energy reserve. One pound of fat represents about 3,500 excess calories.

Between 1985 and 2000, the average daily caloric consumption of Americans rose 12%, the equivalent of about 300 calories, as reported in the U.S. Per Capita Food Supply Trends. Total dietary fat intake remained steady from 1985 to 1999, but jumped 6% in 2000. Another report based on a 2000 study by the American Society for Clinical Nutrition found that an alarming 31% of the calories Americans consume comes from junk food and alcoholic beverages.

Many of these "junk" foods break down quickly to sugar in the blood, drawing some people into a vicious cycle. With more glucose in their blood, the pancreas goes into overdrive to make extra insulin to process all the sugar. As sugar levels drop, people feel sapped of energy and get hungry. That leads to more eating and, ultimately, additional weight gain. In time, this cycle can overwhelm the pancreas and contribute to type-2 diabetes.

Diabetes: A Nationwide Epidemic

Type-2 diabetes, also known as "adult onset diabetes," now afflicts 16 million Americans. Type-2 diabetes makes up 85% of the total cases of diabetes in the United States, with only 10% being type-1, or "juvenile," diabetes. An additional 41 million other Americans have a condition referred to as "pre-diabetes," a known precursor to type-2 diabetes.

Type-1 diabetes is a genetic auto-immune condition in which the pancreas is unable to produce any insulin at all. In most cases, type-1 diabetes develops suddenly in children and adolescents. People with juvenile diabetes are usually thin, and they must take insulin. With type-2 diabetes, the pancreas produces insulin, but the body is unable to regulate the levels of sugar in the blood. Type-2 diabetes typically develops slowly in overweight adults over the age of 40, and can usually be controlled with diet and exercise, though new medications are also now prescribed to help keep blood sugar in balance. When adult-onset diabetes is not kept in check, it can result in a reduction or even a cessation of insulin production in the pancreas, at which point the person must receive insulin.

Shockingly, in the last several years type-2 diabetes has been diagnosed in very young children. Although this form of childhood diabetes most often occurs in adolescents, children as young as four years old have been diagnosed in recent years. But until recently, it was virtually unheard of in children of any age.

As many as 90% of people with adult-onset diabetes, including children and adolescents, are reportedly overweight. For adults, nearly a third (27%) of new cases of type-2 diabetes are attributable to a weight gain of 11 or more pounds. Studies indicate that obesity is the most significant environment influence on the prevalence of type-2 diabetes. Obesity not only is a primary cause of diabetes, it also interferes with the effectiveness of the medications used to treat type-2 diabetes. Talk about a Catch 22.

Diabetes is associated with long-term complications that negatively impact almost every major system in the body. It can cause blindness, heart disease, kidney failure, nerve damage, and stroke, which reduce the quality of life and can lead to death. A study from the Centers for Disease Control estimated that men who are diagnosed with diabetes by age 40 will lose 11 years off their lives and women will lose 14.

Medication alone is usually not enough to control type-2 diabetes and to significantly diminish the risk of impairment resulting from diabetes. The most powerful treatments for adult-onset diabetes—particularly when they are used together—are weight loss and regular exercise.

Other Ill Effects of Obesity

Obesity is a contributing cause—along with physical inactivity, fami-

Symptoms of Diabetes

The following are the common symptoms of diabetes. Not everyone with diabetes will experience all or even most of these symptoms.

- Blurry eyesight
- Dry skin
- Excessive thirst
- Fatigue and sleepiness
- Feeling weak
- Frequent urination (even at night)
- Itchy skin
- Numbness or tingling in feet
- Persistent hunger
- Skin infections
- Slow healing of cuts
- Weight loss

ly history, high blood sugar, high blood pressure, high cholesterol levels, and smoking—of numerous serious medication conditions.

- Arthritis—Hand, hip, back, and knee
- Cancer—Breast, esophagus/gastric, colorectal, endometrial, and kidney (renal)
- Cardiovascular Disease
- Carpal Tunnel Syndrome
- Deep Vein Thrombosis
- Gallbladder Disease
- Gout
- Hypertension—Over 75% of cases directly related to obesity
- Impaired Immune Response
- Impaired Respiratory Function
- Infection—Increased risk of lung (pneumonia), sinus, urinary, and wound infection
- Infertility
- Liver Disease—Cirrhosis, acute hepatitis, nonalcoholic steatohepatitis
- Lower Back Pain

- Pain—Musculoskeletal, joint, foot pain
- Pancreatitis
- Pregnancy
- Complications
- Gestational diabetes, urinary infection, prolonged labor, Cesarean section, toxemia, post-delivery infection
- Sleep Apnea
- Stroke
- Surgical Complications
- Urinary Stress Incontinence

Why are Americans so overweight and suffering the consequences of it? Because we are drowning in calories and starving for exercise. It is time to make a change. Our quality of life and our very lives depend on it. The 10,000-Steps-A-Day Program can help you lose weight and exercise regularly.

The Positive Effects of Exercise

By the time you've reached this point in the book, you're no doubt familiar with the many benefits of being physically active and of walking in particular. To give you even more incentive to get and stay active, here are a few more health-related benefits of exercising regularly:

- A weight loss of as little as 5% of total

FitnessFACT
Four Interlocking Keys to Weight Loss

The National Weight Control Registry maintains a list of about 4,000 people who have lost an average of 67 pounds and kept it off an average of six years. The vast majority of the 4,000 people on the National Weight Control Registry who have lost an average of 67 pounds and kept it off for 6 years have done so through a combination of four strategies:

1. Eating a low-fat diet
2. Rarely missing breakfast
3. Weighing themselves regularly
4. Getting an hour of exercise a day, mostly by walking.

body weight can reduce high blood sugar.

- A weight loss of 10 to 15 pounds will relieve symptoms and can slow progression of arthritis.
- Walking briskly for 1 hour a day can reduce a woman's risk of type-2 diabetes by 50%.
- Walking briskly for 30 minutes 6 times a month can lower the risk of premature death by 44%.
- Walking an hour or more a week can reduce the risk of a first heart attack by 73%.
- Women under age 40 who exercise at least 4 hours per week lessen their risk of breast cancer by up to 58%.
- 45-minutes of moderate to brisk walking will help raise HDL ("good" cholesterol). For every one-point increase in HDL, the risk of heart disease is lowered by 3% in women and by 2% in men.
- A single 30- to 60-minute walk of moderate to brisk intensity can lower triglyceride levels in the

blood by 15 to 40%, and the effects last 36 to 48 hours.
- Exercise can reduce "visceral" fat, even if no weight is lost. Visceral fat is located deep inside the abdominal cavity, surrounding organs, and increases the risk of heart disease, type-2 diabetes, and strokes in middle age.
- Elderly people who have exercised regularly and vigorously all of their lives are 2 to 3 decades younger physically than their contemporaries.
- People who exercise regularly throughout their lives may be at a lower risk of Alzheimers, according to recent studies by the American Academy of Neurology and the University of Cleveland.
- Brisk walkers have a 43% reduced risk of premature death and even occasional moderate walkers have a 29% better chance of living full lives than do sedentary people.

FitnessFACT
Fast Food Nation

In his masterpiece of investigative reporting, Fast Food Nation: The Dark Side of the All-American Meal (Houghton Mifflin), author Eric Schlosser uncovers some startling facts about Americans and their fast food habits.
- Every day about 25% of the U.S. population eats fast food.
- American children now get about 25% of their total vegetable servings in the form of nutrition-less potato chips and French fries.
- The typical teenage boy in the United States now gets about 10% of his daily calories from soda.
- The typical American now consumes approximately three hamburgers and four orders of French fries every week.
- About 90% of American children between the ages of 3 and 9 visit a fast-food burger joint once a month.

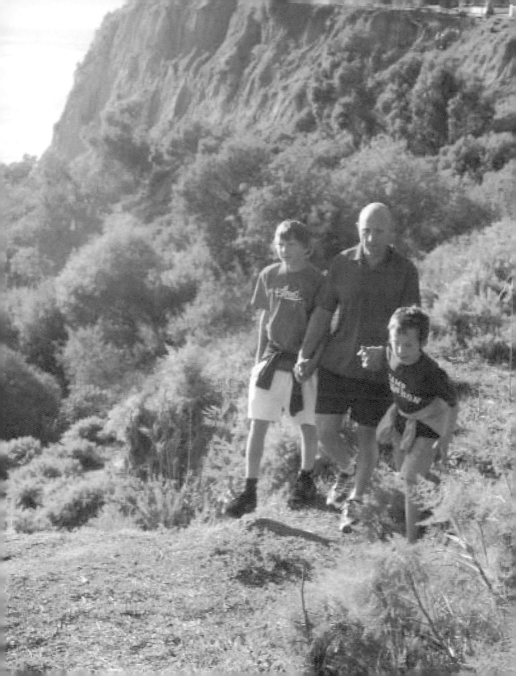

CHAPTER ELEVEN

STEP IT UP

Going for 10,000-Plus

The main objective of the 10,000-Steps-A-Day Program is to help you make regular exercise and healthy eating a routine part of your everyday life. Adopting the healthy habits of walking at least 30 minutes a day and cutting at least 100 calories a day will help you to manage your weight, improve your overall fitness, and decrease your risk of chronic illness.

If you are relatively fit when you begin the 10,000-Steps-A-Day Program, you could well lose a few pounds, shed an inch or two, and tone some of your muscles during the six months of the program. Of course, we hope you will then continue to walk and to eat a balanced diet for many months and years to come, in order to sustain your current weight and level of fitness.

If, on the other hand, you are significantly overweight and/or have been inactive for an extended period of time, you may want to increase your physical activity beyond 10,000 steps a day and to shave additional calories from your daily diet—but only after you've completed both 90-day levels of

FitnessFACT
Thinner-Plus

The main reasons most people start a weight-loss program are to look better and to feel better about themselves, which are perfectly reasonable motivations. Usually, improving their overall fitness and health are secondary motivators, but they are equally important to your health and happiness, particularly over the long run. Here are a few of the most important health benefits of weight loss:

• Lowers elevated blood-sugar (glucose) levels in overweight and obese people with type-2 diabetes.

• Lowers elevated levels of total cholesterol, LDL ("bad") cholesterol, and triglycerides and increases low levels of HDL ("good") cholesterol in overweight and obese people with compromised cholesterol panels (dyslipidemia).

• Lowers elevated blood pressure in overweight and obese people with high blood pressure.

the 10,000-Steps-A-Day Program. As you've seen in Chapter Ten, being overweight puts you at higher risk of numerous serious health problems and early death. It also can diminish your self-esteem and the quality of your life.

Numerous studies have shown that the most effective way to lose weight and keep it off is to do it gradually, by making incremental changes in your eating and physical activity patterns. If you want and need to lose weight, the 10,000-Plus segment of this walking program can help you trim down safely and permanently.

You've Got to Really Move It to Lose It

If you're overweight or obese and want to slim down to a healthy weight, you will need to work up to 12,000 to 15,000 steps a day, the rough equivalent of 60 to 90 minutes worth of moderate-to-

"Sometimes, being pushed to the wall gives the momentum necessary to get over it."

—Peter deJager

brisk walking (6,000 to 9,000 steps) a day. So, if, by the end of the six-month 10,000-Steps-A-Day Program, you are averaging 6,000 steps a day (your new baseline), you would need to add at least another 6,000 steps a day to reach 12,000 steps a day. (For simplicity, you can find your new baseline by adding together your total daily steps for the last 2 weeks of Level 2 and dividing by 14.) If your new baseline is 10,000 steps a day, you would need to add another 2,000 steps a day to reach 12,000 or an additional 5,000 steps a day to reach 15,000.

Remember: You don't need to add all the steps in a single walking or other exercise activity. You can break it up into smaller pieces, of 10 to 30 minutes each.

At the same time, you will need to create an "energy deficit" of 500 to 1,000 calories a day. This does not mean you need to cut 500 to 1,000 calories a day; it means you would need to consume 500 to 1,000 fewer calories than you expend through physical activity, on average, each day. Here's another way to look at creating an energy deficit: A pound of fat equals about 3,500 calories; to lose 1 pound a week, you would need to burn 3,500 more calories than you eat during the week. You can accomplish that by either increasing your physical activity, decreasing your eating, or a

>>**tip**

It's Just Emotions Taking You Over

Substitute emotional walking with emotional eating. Physical activity is an excellent stress-buster. When things start to get to you, rather than reaching for a cookie or indulging in a fat-filled "comfort" food like macaroni and cheese, get up on your feet and take a 10-minute or even a 5-minute walk.

combination of moving more and eating less, which is what most experts and doctors recommend.

Losing 1 to 2 pounds a week over a period of 6 months is a sensible and achievable weigh-loss strategy that is endorsed by the Centers for Disease Control, the U.S. Surgeon General, and virtually all reputable health, nutrition, and weight loss professionals. These same experts recommend that your initial goal should be to reduce your body weight by about 10% of what your weight is at the start of the program. They also say that the 6-month weight-loss program should be immediately followed by a 6-month "maintenance" program, whereby you continue to exercise about 30 minutes a day (or to take 10,000 total steps a day) and to eat a healthy diet.

That is essentially the focus of the 10,000-Plus plan:

If, at the end of your 6-month weight-loss and 6-month maintenance programs, you want to lose additional weight, you can step it up again. Just start a new 6-month program of walking 60 to 90 minutes a day (or taking 12,000 to 15,000 steps a day) and sustaining an energy deficit of about 500 to 1,000 calories a day (or 3,500 calories a week for each pound you want to lose).

For the dietary component of your weight-loss program, reducing both fat and carbohydrates is an effective way to cut calories.

These strategies will help you to achieve and sustain your optimal weight and to improve your health. The 10,000-Plus plan, if completed as outlined and if followed by lifestyle habits of exercising regularly and eating a balanced diet, will also decrease abdominal fat, increase cardiorespiratory fitness, improve muscle tone, and help you live a longer, healthier, happier life.

10,000-Plus: It's a Plan!

Alrighty then! Are you ready to lose weight (and inches) by stepping it up? Good for you! In a nutshell, here is the 10,000-Plus plan:

1. Complete Levels 1 and 2 of the 10,000-Steps-A-Day Program, gradually working toward and getting as close as possible to 10,000 steps a day, while cutting 100 calories a day, preferably foods high in fat and processed sugar. Try to work up to at least 30 minutes of walking per day, and make sure to wear your Step-Counter and to record your step totals in your Daily Step Log every day.

2. Assess your progress, upon completion of the six-month 10,000-Steps-A-Day Program. Did you reach 10,000 steps a day? Were

FitnessFACT

Exercise + Diet + Therapy = Weight Loss for Life

For many people, overeating and obesity are chronic conditions that require a three-pronged approach to weight loss and weight management: (1) moving more, (2) eating less, and (3) resolving the underlying personal reasons compelling that person to eat carelessly and to be sedentary. If you are seriously overweight or obese, or if you feel stuck in a rut and cannot seem to replace unhealthy eating and exercise habits with healthier ones, consider talking with a licensed behavior modification therapist. Try to find a therapist who specializes in weight loss and/or eating disorders. Such a professional can often help you break through the barriers that are preventing you from achieving your weight loss and fitness goals. There also are good self-help books on this subject that can help you get to the bottom of and resolve any "emotional eating" habits you might have.

you able to sustain your highest number of steps for at least a month? Did you cut 100 calories from your daily diet every day or at least most days?

3. Set your 10,000-Plus step goals. Start out at 10,000 to 11,000 steps a day, or 30 to 45 minutes worth of walking, and gradually increase to 12,000 to 15,000 steps a day, or about 60 to 90 minutes worth of walking. Jot down your goal in your Daily Step Log.

4. Set your 10,000-Plus calorie goals. Cut calories, primarily by reducing fat and simple carbohydrates. Create an energy deficit of 500 to 1,000 fewer calories consumed than burned each day (or 3,500 fewer calories consumed than burned per week, for 1 pound of weight loss). Important: Do not create a drastic

energy deficit designed to lose more than 2.5 pounds per week; such a severe energy deficit could harm you and doesn't work anyway, as you usually just regain the weight more quickly.

5. Follow your 10,000-Plus weight-loss plan. Get in your goal of concentrated physical activity every day, starting at 30 to 45 minutes and gradually working up to 60 to 90 minutes a day over the course of 6 months. You can get your steps through walking in combination with any aerobic physical activity (at least 20 minutes of moderate to intense exercise). Also try to increase the steps you take in your everyday life, which count toward your goal of 12,000 to 15,000 totals steps a day, but make sure to get in your daily recommended dose of actual aerobic exercise. Wear your Step-Counter and record your steps in your Daily Step Log. Make sure to follow a low-calorie eating plan and to maintain an adequate energy deficit.

"At times of great stress, it is especially necessary to achieve a complete freeing of the muscles."

—Constantin Stanislavski

6. Follow up with your 10,000-Plus maintenance plan. Tone it down to no fewer than 10,000 to 12,000 steps a day, or 30 to 45 minutes of walking for 6 months. Make sure to follow a low-calorie eating plan and to maintain an adequate energy deficit.

7. Step it up again, if you want to lose additional weight. Start a

second round of your 6-month weight loss plan, followed by another 6-month maintenance plan.

8. Celebrate your accomplishment! Yes, looking and feeling great are their own rewards. But trimming down and improving your fitness is a tremendous achievement that deserves special recognition. So, take the time to revel in your victory. Reward yourself with a new outfit, a romantic weekend with your significant other, a night out on the town with your friends, or anything your heart desires (even a delicious gourmet meal or a small portion of a decadent dessert is fine once in a while). Celebrate you!

CHAPTER TWELVE

THE FINISHING STEP

Body Strengthening and Toning

Congratulations! Assuming that you're several weeks into your 10,000-Steps-A-Day Program by now, you've no doubt succeeded in making regular physical activity a part of your lifestyle. If you're itching to take your new fitness attitude to the next level, you can now add stretching and strength training to your weekly exercise routine to help improve the shape, flexibility, and strength of your body. These simple exercise components will also help you burn extra calories and kick your energy into high gear.

Remember, anytime you start a new exercise program you should check first with your doctor and ease into your new activities. Make sure to also wear your Step-Counter as you do these exercises and to record your total steps in your Daily Log Book. Now, get ready to take the next step.

That's a Stretch

Now that you're strengthening your cardiovascular system and burning more calories with walking, it's time to add stretching to your fitness repertoire. You can add stretching at any point in your 10,000-Steps-A-Day Program, starting with Day One.

According to the American Council on Exercise, stretching regularly will help you enjoy:

• Increased range of motion in your joints and muscles
• Better posture
• Physical and mental relaxation
• Decreased tension and soreness in your muscles

Perform the following stretches after walking or an equivalent physical activity (such as swimming or shooting hoops), when your muscles are warmed up. Move slowly into each stretch, hold for about 10 to 30 seconds without bouncing, and keep breathing. Make sure to back off if it hurts—these stretches shouldn't feel painful.

> **" *Great things are not done by impulse, but by a series of small things brought together.* "**
>
> –Vincent Van Gogh

Arm Cross

Stand with your right arm slightly flexed and positioned horizontally across your body. With your left hand, grasp just above the right elbow, and gently pull your arm across your chest. Repeat with your left arm.

Straddle

Sit on the floor in a "butterfly" position with your knees bent and pointed outward, and with the soles of your feet facing in. Bend from the waist and extend your arms forward. Avoid rounding your shoulders.

Knee Flex

Lying on your back, bring your right leg up by flexing your knee and hip. Gently pull your thigh toward your chest and hold. Now repeat with your left leg.

Wall Stretch

Stand facing a wall with your feet set as wide as your shoulders and your toes about a foot from the wall. Lean forward and put your palms on the wall. Step your right foot back about two feet and flex your left knee. Slowly straighten your right leg and lower your heel to the floor. Repeat with your left foot back.

Save Your Strength

After our mid- to late-twenties, we gradually lose muscle as we age. Because muscle burns calories for fuel, the more muscle you have and the more you exercise, the higher your metabolism, even when you're not exercising. As you lose muscle, you'll find it more difficult to lose weight and to keep it off.

That's where strength training can help. Sometimes referred to

> **" The sum of the whole is this:
> Walk and be happy; walk and
> be healthy. The best way to
> lengthen out our days is to walk
> steadily and with a purpose. "**
>
> *–Charles Dickens*

as "weightlifting" and "resistance training," this form of exercise uses hand weights, elastic straps, machines, or your own body weight to provide resistance during exercise. By doing strength training exercises regularly—two to four times a week—you can help counteract muscle loss and even increase muscle size, which helps to stoke your metabolism and burn more calories throughout the day.

Resistance training can also make it easier to perform everyday activities, such as climbing stairs and carrying groceries, and make your bones healthier. In a study of postmenopausal women, participants who did strength-training in combination with their regular exercise activities for a year increased their bone density by 1 percent, while those who did not and were sedentary lost 2 percent.

Strength-training is beneficial at any age, not just middle age. Obviously, younger adults from age 18 through their 20s, 30s, and 40s can reap significant benefits from building and strengthening muscles, bones, and joints, which is precisely what strength-training is designed to do. What many people don't realize is that strength-training is beneficial to people far beyond middle age, straight through their golden years.

Think it's too late for you to start lifting weights? Consider the research that's been done on seniors. In a study of 90-year-olds at Tufts University, eight weeks of resistance training resulted in a whopping strength gain of 174%, on average. If a 94-year-old can double his or her strength, imagine what you can do!

To get you started, we've designed a beginning strength training program that targets muscles throughout your body, three days a week.

Start-Up Strength-Training Routine

Do the following strength-training exercises three times a week. For simplicity, we've scheduled these sessions for Monday, Wednesday, and Friday, but you can schedule them for any three days of the week you prefer—just make sure to include at least 1 day off and no more than 2 days off in between sessions.

Perform 8 to 12 repetitions of each exercise and then repeat the whole set a second time. Use enough weight so that the last repetition feels difficult but doesn't overstrain muscles or throw off your form. Always lift slowly; never swing or yank the weight or resistance strap.

You'll find instructions for each exercise as well as helpful photos on pages 233 through 241

Calorie-Burning Overdrive

After you've been on the walking program and stretching and

Monday	Wednesday	Abdominal crunch
Lunge	Squat	Back extension
Leg curl	Leg curl	
Barbell or machine chest	Dumbbell or machine	**Friday**
press	chest press	Repeat Monday or
Seated row	Lat pull-down	Wednesday's routine
Overhead press	Side lateral raise with	
Dumbbell curl	dumbbells	
Abdominal crunch	Overhead tricep dumbbell	
Back extension	press	

doing strength-training for about eight weeks, you can increase the intensity (and calorie burning power) of your walking by adding hand weights or intervals to your walks or by jogging.

Hand Weights. Holding light dumbbells while walking will increase your calorie burn and strengthen your shoulder muscles. Use 1-pound or 2-pound weights; don't use a higher weight than that. Never use hand weights while walking if you have problems with your back, shoulders, wrists, or knees or if you have high blood pressure (gripping can raise it). Weighted gloves—starting at about $10—can be a safer option, because you're not as likely to drop them on your toes or shins. Use a moderate (natural) arm swing with your elbows bent to about 90 degrees, moving from your shoulders, not your elbows. Do not swing too far or fast. Your hands should rise to about chest level.

Intervals. Another way to increase your calorie burn is by including higher intensity intervals during your walks— walking at a very fast pace for 2 to 5 minutes, then slowing to an easier pace for 2 to 5 minutes. Initially, repeat the fast-slow intervals twice in the middle of your walk, eventually working up to 6 to 8 intervals per session. When you quicken your pace, make sure not to over-stride or lock your knees, which can lead to injury.

Jogging. If you've been thinking about joining those runners you see out during your walks, it might be time to break into a jog. Start by including two sets of 2-minute jogs in the middle of your walk, with 5 minutes of brisk walking in between. As the weeks go by, gradually increase the amount of time you're jogging, so that after about four months you're able to walk for 5 minutes at a moderate to brisk pace, run for 20 minutes, walk briskly for 5 minutes, run for another 20, and finish with 5 minutes of moderate walking (to cool down).

Joining Up

Joining a gym gives you access to lots of fitness equipment; specialized classes, such as kickboxing; and personal trainers, who can help set you up on a training program to match your goals. Before signing on the dotted line, however, carefully evaluate the gyms in your area before making your selection. The features and equipment offered as well as the quality of the facility, programs, and trainers can vary greatly. With more than 26,000 fitness clubs nationwide, though, you are sure to find one that suits your personal needs and preferences.

Look for a club that's close to your home or work. If it's out of the way, you'll be less likely to go regularly. The training staff should be certified by a nationally recognized organization. Some of the more well-known and credible groups include the American Council on Exercise (ACE), the American College of Sports Medicine (ACSM), the National Strength and Conditioning Association (NSCA), and the National Academy of Sports Medicine (NASM).

Questions to ask when checking out a fitness club include:

• Does the staff participate in ongoing professional training?
• Are staff members trained in CPR, the use of automated external defibrillators and first aid?
• Will I be given a pre-exercise health screening?
• Does the club offer a trial membership?

Strength Training Exercises

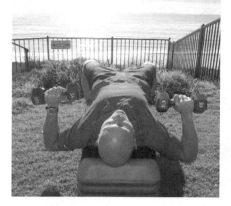 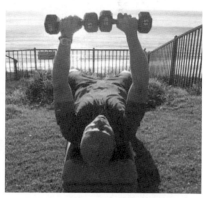

Dumbbell Flat Bench Press

1. Lie face up on a flat bench with your feet on the ground and a dumbbell in each hand.

2. Bend your arms and position your hands at your armpits with your palms facing toward your legs. You should feel a slight stretch in your chest and shoulders.

3. Raise your dumbbells together over your chest while extending your arms and rotate your wrists to face each other.

4.. Return to the starting position, aiming your elbows downward and back slightly.

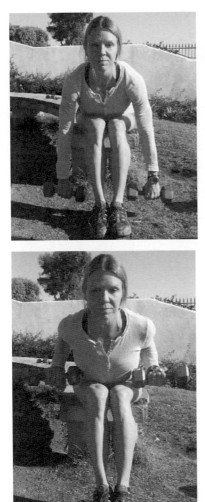

Seated Dumbbell Back Lateral

1. Sit on the end of a flat bench with a dumbbell in each hand down at your side and your palms facing backward.

2. Lean forward as much as possible and allow the dumbbells to come together just above your feet.

3. Pull the dumbbells up as you lift your elbows upward and back along the side of your body, while squeezing your shoulder blades together.

4. Rotate your palms so that they face inward at the end of the movement.

5. Return your hands slowly to the position just above your feet.

236

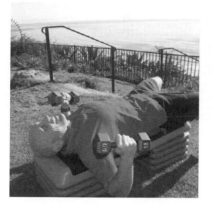
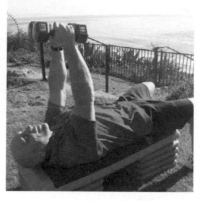

Dumbbell Fly

1. Lie face up on a flat bench with your feet on the floor and a dumbbell in each hand.

2. Begin with your arms slightly bent and directly out to the side, palms up and the dumbbells in line with your chest. Allow the dumbbells to push your arms down so that you feel a slight stretch.

3. In an arc-like motion, bring the dumbbells together over your upper chest with palms facing each other.

4. Return to the starting position slowly.

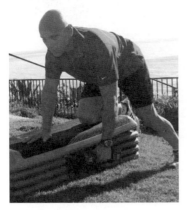

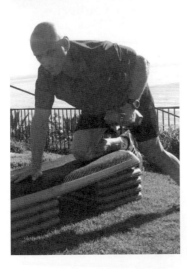

One-Arm Dumbbell Row

1. Position the body over a flat bench with one knee on the bench and the hand of the same side on the front of the bench so your back is flat.

2. Your opposite foot should be securely on the floor.

3. Hold a dumbbell in your free hand and allow the arm to extend fully straight down with your palm facing your foot.

4. Pull the dumbbell upward to the hip while rotating the palm inward. Point the elbow as far upward as possible.

5. Return slowly to the starting position.

6. Repeat on right and left sides.

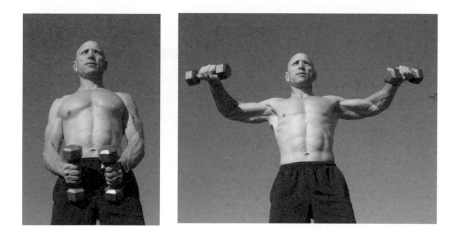

Lateral Raise

1. Hold a dumbbell in each hand, with your palms facing inward.

2. Your feet should be planted firmly about shoulder width apart but with a slight bend in the knees. Again, the chin is up and the chest is out, with a slight arch in the back as you bend forward twenty or thirty degrees at the waist.

3. Bending your elbows slightly, raise the dumbbells to your side to just above shoulder height, "leading" with the elbows.

4. Pause at the top and then lower them.

5. Repeat for the next rep.

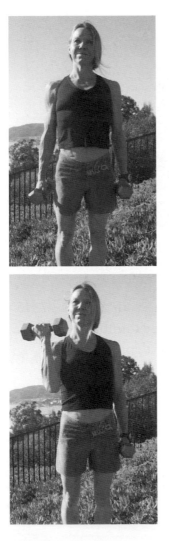

Alternate Dumbbell Curl

1. Stand with your feet at a comfortable width and your knees slightly bent.

2. With your arms at your sides, hold the dumbbells so that your palms face the body.

3. Keep your back straight and bend one arm, raising the dumbbell to the shoulder and rotating the palm upward.

4. Return the arm slowly, and as you near the starting position, begin the same movement with your other arm.

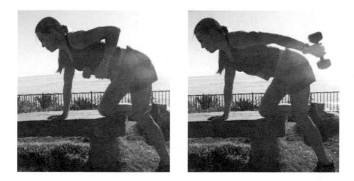

Triceps Kickback

1. Position the body over a flat bench with one knee on the bench and the hand of the same side on the front of the bench so that the back is parallel to the ground.

2. Your opposite foot should be securely on the floor.

3. Hold a dumbbell with your free hand and position your upper arm parallel to the floor and braced against the body.

4. Bend your arm fully with your palm facing inward, then extend the dumbbell backward using your forearm, moving only at the elbow until your arm is straight.

5. Return the arm to the bent position.

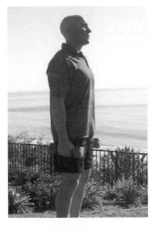

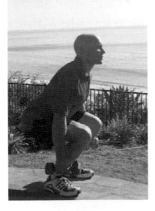

Dumbbell Squats

1. Stand with your feet shoulder width apart and your toes pointed out slightly.

2. Hold a dumbbell in each hand at shoulder height or down to your sides.

3. With your back erect, bend both your knees simultaneously as you lower yourself until your upper thigh is parallel to the floor.

4. Return to the upright position without locking your knees.

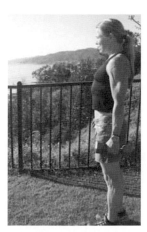
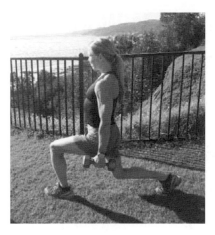

Walking Lunges

1. Begin by holding dumbbells in each hand and standing erect.

2. Take a large step forward and lower your body by bending both knees. The knee on your forward leg should stay above the ankle, while the rear knee nearly touches the floor.

3. Return to the upright position as if you were walking forward. In other words, let the trailing leg catch up.

4. Press with the heel of your front leg as you come up, and squeeze the buttocks as you bring your legs together.

5. Repeat the movement with opposite leg.

Step Goals Worksheet

Baseline: _____ steps

Level One Goals

90-Day Goal: _____ steps

	Duration	Exercise Steps per day	Total Steps per day (baseline + exercise)
Week 1			
Week 2			
Week 3			
Week 4			
Week 5			
Week 6			
Week 7			
Week 8			
Week 9			
Week 10			
Week 11			
Week 12			

Step Goals Worksheet

Baseline: _____ steps

Level Two Goals

90-Day Goal: _____ steps

	Duration	Exercise Steps per day	Total Steps per day (baseline + exercise)
Week 13			
Week 14			
Week 15			
Week 16			
Week 17			
Week 18			
Week 19			
Week 20			
Week 21			
Week 22			
Week 23			
Week 24			

Step Activity Planner

Level One

90-Day Goal: _____ steps

Week 1	Activity Time	Duration
Mon.		
Tues.		
Wed.		
Thur.		
Fri.		
Sat.		
Sun.		

Week 2	Activity Time	Duration
Mon.		
Tues.		
Wed.		
Thur.		
Fri.		
Sat.		
Sun.		

Week 3	Activity Time	Duration
Mon.		
Tues.		
Wed.		
Thur.		
Fri.		
Sat.		
Sun.		

Week 4	Activity Time	Duration
Mon.		
Tues.		
Wed.		
Thur.		
Fri.		
Sat.		
Sun.		

Week 5	Activity Time	Duration
Mon.		
Tues.		
Wed.		
Thur.		
Fri.		
Sat.		
Sun.		

Week 6	Activity Time	Duration
Mon.		
Tues.		
Wed.		
Thur.		
Fri.		
Sat.		
Sun.		

Step Activity Planner Level One

Week 7	Activity Time	Duration
Mon.		
Tues.		
Wed.		
Thur.		
Fri.		
Sat.		
Sun.		

Week 8	Activity Time	Duration
Mon.		
Tues.		
Wed.		
Thur.		
Fri.		
Sat.		
Sun.		

Week 9	Activity Time	Duration
Mon.		
Tues.		
Wed.		
Thur.		
Fri.		
Sat.		
Sun.		

Week 10	Activity Time	Duration
Mon.		
Tues.		
Wed.		
Thur.		
Fri.		
Sat.		
Sun.		

Week 11	Activity Time	Duration
Mon.		
Tues.		
Wed.		
Thur.		
Fri.		
Sat.		
Sun.		

Week 12	Activity Time	Duration
Mon.		
Tues.		
Wed.		
Thur.		
Fri.		
Sat.		
Sun.		

Step Activity Planner Level Two

Week 13	Activity Time	Duration
Mon.		
Tues.		
Wed.		
Thur.		
Fri.		
Sat.		
Sun.		

Week 14	Activity Time	Duration
Mon.		
Tues.		
Wed.		
Thur.		
Fri.		
Sat.		
Sun.		

Week 15	Activity Time	Duration
Mon.		
Tues.		
Wed.		
Thur.		
Fri.		
Sat.		
Sun.		

Week 16	Activity Time	Duration
Mon.		
Tues.		
Wed.		
Thur.		
Fri.		
Sat.		
Sun.		

Week 17	Activity Time	Duration
Mon.		
Tues.		
Wed.		
Thur.		
Fri.		
Sat.		
Sun.		

Week 18	Activity Time	Duration
Mon.		
Tues.		
Wed.		
Thur.		
Fri.		
Sat.		
Sun.		

Step Activity Planner Level Two

Week 19	Activity Time	Duration
Mon.		
Tues.		
Wed.		
Thur.		
Fri.		
Sat.		
Sun.		

Week 20	Activity Time	Duration
Mon.		
Tues.		
Wed.		
Thur.		
Fri.		
Sat.		
Sun.		

Week 21	Activity Time	Duration
Mon.		
Tues.		
Wed.		
Thur.		
Fri.		
Sat.		
Sun.		

Week 22	Activity Time	Duration
Mon.		
Tues.		
Wed.		
Thur.		
Fri.		
Sat.		
Sun.		

Week 23	Activity Time	Duration
Mon.		
Tues.		
Wed.		
Thur.		
Fri.		
Sat.		
Sun.		

Week 24	Activity Time	Duration
Mon.		
Tues.		
Wed.		
Thur.		
Fri.		
Sat.		
Sun.		

Daily Step Log

Baseline

	Mon.	Tue.	Wed.	Thu.	Fri.	Sat.	Sun.	Total Steps (wk)
Week 1								
Week 2								
Total Baseline Steps								

(add Week 1 and Week 2 totals)

_____ (Total Baseline Steps) ÷ 14 (Days) = _____ (Baseline)

10,000-Steps-A-Day Program
Level One

	Mon.	Tue.	Wed.	Thu.	Fri.	Sat.	Sun.	Total Steps (wk)
Week 1								
Week 2								
Week 3								
Week 4								
Week 5								
Week 6								
Week 7								
Week 8								
Week 9								
Week 10								
Week 11								
Week 12								

10,000-Steps-A-Day Program
Level Two

	Mon.	Tue.	Wed.	Thu.	Fri.	Sat.	Sun.	Total Steps (wk)
Week 13								
Week 14								
Week 15								
Week 16								
Week 17								
Week 18								
Week 19								
Week 20								
Week 21								
Week 22								
Week 23								
Week 24								

10,000-Plus Program
Level One

	Mon.	Tue.	Wed.	Thu.	Fri.	Sat.	Sun.	Total Steps (wk)
Week 1								
Week 2								
Week 3								
Week 4								
Week 5								
Week 6								
Week 7								
Week 8								
Week 9								
Week 10								
Week 11								
Week 12								

10,000-Plus Program
Level Two

	Mon.	Tue.	Wed.	Thu.	Fri.	Sat.	Sun.	Total Steps (wk)
Week 13								
Week 14								
Week 15								
Week 16								
Week 17								
Week 18								
Week 19								
Week 20								
Week 21								
Week 22								
Week 23								
Week 24								